Introduction

This text was condensed from orthopaedic textbooks, papers, online sources and revision notes to create a questions and answers bank with easily citable classic orthopaedic evidence designed for testing and revision practice for the viva element of the FRCS Orth exam (United Kingdom). The general themes and topics are readily transferable to any orthopaedic postgraduate viva exam.

Geraint Williams MBchB FRCS Orth

Contents

Chapter 1:   **Adult Reconstruction Hip**

Chapter 2:   **Adult Reconstruction Knee**

Chapter 3:   **Statistics, Biomaterials & Physics**

Chapter 4:   **Basic science**

Chapter 5:   **Upper Limb Trauma**

Chapter 6:   **Lower Limb Trauma**

Chapter 7:   **Foot & Ankle**

Chapter 8:   **Hand & Microsurgery**

Chapter 9:   **Shoulder & Elbow**

Chapter 10:   **Paediatric Genetics & Dysplasia**

Chapter 11:   **Neuromuscular Paediatrics**

Chapter 12:   **Paediatric Trauma**

Chapter 13:   **Paediatric Lower Limb**

Chapter 14:   **Pathology**

Chapter 15:   **Adult Spine**

Chapter 1: Adult Reconstruction Hip

Q1. Tell me the difference between apparent and true leg length inequality?

Apparent is the sum of true shortening plus any shortening caused by fixed deformity (minus compensatory movement / tilting, foot equinus). **True** is the actual bone length difference.

Q2. Give me the arterial blood supply of the hip?

Profunda femoris - comes off the lateral side of femoral artery passing deep behind adductor longus (femoral artery stays anterior to it). Then gives off perforators winding around the femur passing into all compartments after the two main branches are given off (below).

Medial femoral circumflex artery (2 branches) – crosses anterior to pectineus and iliopsoas to lie at boarder of adductor longus – passes between this and magnus to the back of the thigh (no intermuscular septum medially) where it divides at the interval between magnus and quadratus femoris to **ascending** (up) and **transverse** branches becomes part of the **cruciate anastomosis**.

Lateral femoral circumflex artery (3 branches) – passes onto the rectus femoris after leaving femoral triangle. Gives off the **ascending** branch passing up between Sartorius and TFL (to be divided in the anterior approach to the hip) up and onto joint capsule. **Transverse** branch to joins the transverse branch of the medial circumflex at the **cruciate** anastomosis and the **descending** branch between vastus lateralis and intermedius.

Cruciate anastomosis comprises the ascending branch of 1st perforating artery, the descending branch of the inferior gluteal artery and the transverse branches of the medial and lateral femoral circumflex arteries.

Q3. Which structures form the femoral triangle?

Superior: inguinal ligament.
Medial: adductor longus.
Floor: adductor longus and iliopsoas.
Lateral: sartorius.
Roof: fascia lata.

Q4. Tell me about piriformis syndrome?

Sciatic nerve entrapment at the level of the ischial tuberosity. Occurs anterior to the piriformis muscle or posterior to the inferior gemellus obturator internus complex. Caused by bipartite piriformis, aneurysms (inferior gluteal artery), tumor or variations in the nerves path. FAIR test flexion adduction int rotation (places the nerve under tension). Treatment should be non-operative, injections, stretching with muscle release only in refractory cases.

Q5. What causes a 'snapping hip'?

Can be **external** due to ITB on the greater trochanter, iliopsoas sliding over the femoral head or a prominent iliopectineal ridge, osteophytes on the lesser trochanter or lesser trochanter bursa iliopsoas. Or **internal** due to loose bodies inside the joint, internal synovial chondromatosis or labral tears. Treat the problem via excision of the bursa ITB Z plasty, release of the iliopsoas tendon or hip arthroscopy.

Q6. Tell me how you would diagnose hip impingement?

Usually a combination of the two types (80%): **Cam** type in young men often secondary to an old SUFE and **pincer** type in middle age ladies. Suspect cam lesion on a false profile view showing small head neck ratio and lateral hip radiograph with an alpha angle of 63 deg for head sphericity. Diagnose pincer impingement with cross over sign on radiographs and a centre edge ankle of >40 degrees (angles are controversial).

Q7. You are planning a hip arthroscopy, where would you place portals?

- **Anterior lateral** over a guidewire 2cm superior to the anterior third of the trochanter.
- **Anterior portal** under image guidance with hip flexed and internal rotation to loosen capsule, 2cm superior and 2cm anterior to the anterior superior boarder of the trochanter (viewing portal).
- **Posterior portal** 2cm posterior to the trochanter
- **Set up** requires a post and traction table 50lbs of traction
- **Complications:** pudendal nerve injury most common on the post and peroneal nerve injury (traction neuropraxia), superior gluteal nerve injury from anterior lateral portal, posterior and lateral portal put sciatic nerve at risk. Anterior portal places femoral neurovascular bundle and lateral femoral cutaneous nerves at risk.

Q8. List me the biomechanical goals of arthroplasty/osteotomy?

- Restore mechanical axis
- Prevent abnormal moments about a joint & uneven contact forces with cuts
- Preserve level of joint
- Balance ligaments
- Rigid fixation for longevity

Q9. Which factors can accelerate total hip replacement aseptic loosening?

- Thickness of poly
- Implantation / cementing technique
- Geometry
- Sterilization
- Conformity

- Backside wear
- Position of implant (edge loading & smaller contact areas)
- Unbalanced or any feature causing asymmetrical loading
- Patient factors: age, gender, OA vs RA, trauma, DDH, Perthes

Q10. You're planning to revise a THR what kit / planning do you need to consider?

- Plan surgical approach
- Discuss with colleges
- Pre-op tests RBC cell saver
- Bone graft
- Large prosthetic inventory, know implant to be removed
- Angiography for intra pelvic cement or pre-op CT
- Stem extraction equipment, pelvic recon cages, trochanteric fixation, cement extraction hardware, light, drills, osteotomies, flexi drills / reamers

Q11. How can you treat a recurrent THR dislocation?

- Bracing for 3 months, around 1/3 of patients will be successful
- After third dislocation = revise according to why you think its dislocating
- Larger femoral head **(Berry, JBJS)**
- Soft tissue repair posterior capsule **(Polici, CORR)**
- Trochanteric advancement **(Eklund, J Arthroplasty)**
- Constrained component **(Goets, JBJS)**
- Revise to a bi polar **(Parvisi, JBJS)**
- Revise implant position / increased offset

Q12. How do you grade quality of cementation?

Barrack (JBJS) Grades of femoral cementing 12-year review

A – Total white out

B – Near complete filling (some demarcation with defects less than 50%)

C1 – More than 50% demarcation

C2 – Either prosthesis is touching the bone or cement mantel <1mm at any point

D – Gross voids. **Types D and C = early failure**

Q13. *What is loosening?*

Radiographic criteria described by **Harris**

DEFINATE
- **Progressive** lucency at cement bone /cement implant, implant bone interface
- **Fracture** of cement mantel / component or migration of component
- **Debonding** lucency at metal cement interface (usually at **Gruen** zone 1) = in Charnley this is abnormal subsidence of the component into the cement but this is normal in an Exeter hip.

Q14. *What indicates a stable hip on radiographs?*

- Absence of radiolucency
- Spot welds
- Proximal stress shielding

Q15. *Alternative causes of lucency or bone loss?*

- Non-filling at time of surgery
- Adaptive remodelling with formation of neo cortex (will remain the same over time)
- Infection
- Loosening
- Stress shielding

Q16. *What types of mechanical wear can you describe?*

Type 1 – between articulating surfaces as you would expect
Type 2 – articulating part wear against non-articulating component
Type 3 – 3rd body wear
Type 4 – between two non-weight bearing surfaces (implant neck against acetabular edge)

Q17. *How do femoral stems fail?*

Gruen's (JBJS) modes of stem failure:

1a. **Pistoning** of just implant
1b. **Pistoning** of the implant and cement with it
2. **Middle stem pivot** (Catherine wheel – fixed in the middle)
3. **Calcar pivot** (fixed at the top but mobile at the bottom)
4. **Cantilever bending** (fixed at the bottom but mobile at the top)

Q18. *Tell me about hip resurfacing? Isn't this contraindicated?*

Answer: No, it can be suitable for young patients and dysplastic hips but does expose the patient to different risks such as

- Neck fracture (2%, 4% in coxa vara),
- Revision rate is 1.5% vs 0.3% for THR in 1st year according to NJR
- Alternative metal ion problems
- Increased rate of heterotopic ossification
- Pseudo-tumour and ALVAL risks

Q19. *What are the contraindications for resurfacing?*

- Leg length deficiency - *LLD* (will not correct)

- Large cysts and bone loss
- Metal hypersensitivity
- Renal function problems
- Osteoporosis
- Grossly abnormal femoral geometry (increased wear rate)
- Inflammatory arthritis
- Female (increases all risks – 5x cup failure, 2x fracture risk, higher ALVAL risk
- Smaller patients where you anticipate a head size less than 46mm (higher risk as for females and increases risk of ALVAL – **aseptic lymphocytic vasculitis associated lesions,** pseudo tumours

Q20. What is the MHRA (United Kingdom), what do they say about metal on metal hips?

MHRA guidelines - *Medicine healthcare products regulatory agency*

Look for these major issues regarding the implant you are dealing with:

- **S**ymptomatic   = not good
- **H**ead size 36mm and above   = not good
- **I**ons: Co Cr   = not good
- **T**ype of implant   = THR bad (resurfacing is ok)

MRI or ultrasound looking for **ALVAL** / pseudotumor / lysis if any of the above.

Fluid collections alone can be watched. Standard follow up if none of the above an issue.

Follow up and 2nd blood test always after the first 3 months. Looking for change in levels, any change then consider more imaging or revision if symptomatic.

Q21. Tell me about cement containing antibiotics?

- Palacos with gentamycin is the NJR favourite (0.5g - 2g per 40g mix) high viscosity
- 12.5g gentamycin is the max dose per 40g mix
- More than 4.5g per 40g mix will weaken cements mechanical properties

Q22. Does the British Hip Society have guidelines in respect to total hip replacement?

- Suggest 20-minute minimum time for consultation initially
- Decision to perform THR should be made by someone with CCT
- Decision should be clinical not based on scoring systems or xrays
- Patients should be told the risk of death within 30 days is 1 in 500
- Ultra clean air theatre, antibiotic loaded cement should be used
- Agree that **WHO** check in should be observed
- Suggest implant selection should be guided by **ODEP** (orthopaedic data evaluation panel) **10a** implants should be followed up 1 yr 7yr then 3 yearly minimum

Q23. Do NICE have anything to say in respect to arthroplasty?

- Use ODEP rated products eg:
- **CORAIL stem** HA coated titanium alloy stem **ODEP 10A**
- **EXETER V40** Orthinox (low corrosion stainless steel) **ODEP 10A**
- **Anticoagulate** for TKR 14days THR 28 days

Q24. What is the UK national joint registry?

- Set up 2002 to monitor implant performance provide feedback

- Revision rates for implant types eg cemented outperform hybrid which outperform uncemented
- Provides reasons for revision: Dislocation (top reason), aseptic loosening, infection, pain, lysis, fracture (least common).

Q25. Can you classify dysplasia in relation to the hip?

Crowe classification of hip dysplasia: two femoral head factors
1) **Proximal displacement**: 10%, 10-15%, 15-20%, >20% (types 1-4)
2) **Subluxation**: < 50%, 50-75%, 75-100%, >100% (types 1-4)

Q26. When might you suspect hip dysplasia on radiographs?

- Decreased **sphericity** of femoral head
- Acetabular **crossover** sign (change in acetabular version)
- Changes in head neck **offset**
- **Protrusio**
- False profile view can show a lateral centre edge angle **<20deg** = dysplasia sign
- **Tonnis angle increased** = inclination of the weight bearing zone – line from horizontal to the medial sourcil to the lateral most weight bearing point usually should be <**10 deg**, if more then it's a sign of dysplasia.

Q27. How can you treat hip dysplasia with no osteoarthritis surgically?

PAO (**Ganz** or **Bernese** with 3-4screws – leaves a sliver of posterior column intact to maintain stability) +/- femoral osteotomy for symptomatic dysplasia with a congruent joint and no arthritis. Alternative is a Shelf or Chiari osteotomy for sublux hip, hip resurfacing or THR.

Q28. Your planning to revise an implant with significant bone loss around the femoral stem and acetabulum, are there any classification you can use to guide treatment?

Paproski classification acetabular bone loss:
1   Cavitatory defect
2a   Superior bone lysis but **rim intact**
2b   Absent superior rim (**segmental defect**) superior lateral migration
2c   Destruction of medial wall and teardrop (**migrations <2cm**)
3a   Defuse bone loss around superior rim **10am – 2pm**, superolateral migration **>2cm**
3b   Defuse bone loss **9am – 5pm** and superior-medial migration so **will have pelvic discontinuity** as cup has moved **medially >2cm**

Paproski classification femoral bone loss:
1   Minimal metaphyseal
2   Extensive metaphyseal loss
3a   Diaphyseal bone loss but **3cm intact** cortical bone before isthmus
3b   Diaphyseal bone loss < **3cm** cortical bone before isthmus
4   Extensive mid diaphyseal bone loss **no support here**

Options depend on bone loss, you must reconstruct and or bypass defective area:

- Can impaction bone graft and cage (**Sherurs, JBJS**)
- **Type 4** requires **step cut** allograft-prothesis composite or **mega prosthesis**
- **Avoid** cemented stems unless irritated bone or v low demand patients
- Consider larger cups, allograft and **Tantalum** augments (**Paproski, JBJS**)

Q29. What's a snapping ilio psoas tendon?

This is a sign of 'external impingement' causing pain as the tendon snaps over anterior structures. The provocation test is with hip extension and internal rotation from a flexed and externally rotated position (*takes tension off then put the tension on*). **Opposite of the internal impingement 'McCarthy sign'.**

Q30. What are the special issues when planning to replace a rheumatoid hip?

- Skin, C spine, TMJ and soft tissues
- Arthrodesis/osteotomy are contra indicated (healing)
- Protrusio = difficult dislocation abnormal cup
- Osteopenic bone may require grafting
- Infection rate is double
- Biology prevents bone remodelling / in / on growth
- Femoral neck is more anteverted and valgus
- Higher revision rate in younger patients (up to 50% at 5yrs in some series)

Q31. What are the special issues when planning to replace the hip in a patient with ankylosing spondylitis?

- Spinal deformity (anaesthetic problem and LLD – if fixed pelvic obliquity)
- Infection and heterotopic ossification risks increased
- Dislocation risk increased, usually anterior due to prior FFD and anteverted acetabulum
- Increased wear rates as younger patients.
- Always consider bilateral THR as the FFD will recur in the operated hip unless you do the other within 2 months.
- THR usually improves back pain (positional).

Q32. Position of hip arthrodesis and why?

- 25 degrees of flexion, which allows the hip to swing efficiently during gait
- 5 degrees of adduction, and 5 degrees of external rotation; this positioning maximizes gait efficiency and also allows the patient to stand appropriately during stance phases of gait.
- Fusion position will minimise need for lumbar spine / other side knee motion
- Less flexion makes sitting more difficult
- More adduction makes female intercourse / urination a problem
- **Methods: AO cobra plate** (disrupts hip abductors extra articular technique). **Trans articular** slide screw into superior acetabulum (long lever arm gives a non-union risk) and **combined approaches** intra and extra articular fusion with bone graft

Q33. Tell me the contraindications to hip arthrodesis and its outcomes?

Contraindications: Higher BMI, systemic arthritis, contralateral hip spine or same side knee disease deformity or instability, requires **30%** more exergy to walk

Outcome: 15 years after surgery arthritis found in lumbar spine (>50-100%), ipsilateral knee and contralateral knee (>50%), and contralateral hip (>25%-50%).

Revision of arthrodesis to THR – takes 2yrs to regain full abductor strength. High complication rate: 2-15% infection, up to 6% dislocation, nerve injury up to 13%, 33% revision rate at 10 years. Absent abductor function is a contraindication for conversion.

Q34. How have we progressed in respect to cementation techniques?

1st Generation   Finger pack, no plug, sharp corners, narrow borders, stainless-steel

2nd Generation implants	Plugging, lavage, gun, super alloy, smooth
3rd Generation	Vacuum porosity reduction, surface modifications of implants, pressurized PMMA application, stem centralization proximally and distally

Q35. What are the ideal conditions for bone integration for non-cemented implants?

- Optimum pore size 150micro meters
- Porosity 50%
- Maximum micromotion 150 microns
- Bone implant distance 50 micrometres or less

Q36. What kinds of nerve injury can occur when performing THR?

- **Risk:** 0.5-3% primary, 7.5% in revision
- Most common injury is to the **peroneal branch of the sciatic nerve** followed by the femoral nerve.
- The **obturator nerve** can be injured during cemented THAs when cement escapes the confines of the pelvis.
- Lateral femoral cutaneous nerve can be injured via pressure from pelvic positioners
- **Risk Factors:** Female, DDH, LLD, small patients, pre-existing lumbar disease or neuropathy, post traumatic arthritis, posterior approach, uncemented implants
- 90% recover but usually incomplete

Q37. What are the risk factors for heterotopic ossification?

Risk factors: males, hypertrophic arthritis, ankylosing spondylitis, (DISH), posttraumatic OA, hip fusion conversions, Parkinson's disease, excessive osteophytosis, or enthesopathy, anterior and lateral approaches to the hip, length of the surgical procedure and the extent of soft tissue disruption inflicted during surgery.

Brookers grading:
I.   Islands of bone within the soft tissues
II.   Bone off the pelvis or proximal end of femur with at least 1-cm gap
III.   Bone off the pelvis or the proximal end of femur with less than 1-cm gap
IV.   Bone connecting the pelvis and femur (ankylosis)

Treatment: grade **III** or **IV** disease that **restricts motion** are generally good candidates for surgical removal 1 year after THA followed by 7-8 grey single dose radiotherapy within 24 hours after surgery or indomethacin 75 mg/day for 6 weeks postoperatively.

Q38. *What is radial clearance?*

Radial clearance – the difference between the radius of the cup contact area and head (THR). If radius of the head the larger, bearing contact is **equatorial** = high frictional torque and no space for lubricant if smaller than the cup, bearing contact is **polar** = high radial clearance high friction stress and wear. The *optimum* design is polar contact with high bearing conformity (typically <**150** μm of radial clearance is ideal). The low radial clearance is still enough to allow ingress and egress of the lubricant into the bearing.

Q39. *Tell me about the different mechanical wear patterns associated with different bearing combinations?*

Stripe wear occurs with **hard-on-hard bearing** - crescent-shaped line that forms on a femoral head & cup (vertical orientation of cup increases this). **Ceramic** surfaces suffer from **grain pullout**. With a metal surface, **abrasive wear** is common. With poly **adhesive** and **abrasive** wear occurs (hard on soft bearing couple).

Q40. *What are the changes associated with avascular necrosis of the hip?*

Ficats radiographic stages
Stage 1 MRI changes
Stage 2 sclerosis and crescent sign (pre-collapse)
Stage 3 head flattening (collapse)
Stage 4 arthritis on both sides of the joint

Q41. *How can you treat AVN of the hip?*

- Observation will fail 80% collapse further by 4yrs (**Ohzono**).
- Use of alendronate prolongs survival without surgery (prevents collapse)
- Oxygen therapy for 100 days in stage 1 increases survival
- Core decompression (**Mont**), 2/3 do well +/- tantalum rod +/- graft (vascular)
- Trapdoor procedure (**Mont**), Grades III/IV (**Ficat**) 2/3 good results
- Muscle pedicle grafts or rectus femoris graft.
- Osteotomy – angular or rotational for younger patients (avoid in alcohol / steroid), Ficat stage II/III/IV
- Hemi caps
- THR
- Resurface
- Arthrodesis.

Natural history: smaller anterior medial lesions = unlikely to progress, (**Mont**) pooled analysis of 27 studies THR failure 10-50% at 5yrs if performed for AVN. Prompting use of core decompression techniques with 5-year survival without THR depending on stage. Stage 1 >80% 2 > 60% 3 > 40% 5-year survival without THR.

Q42. *Tell me about protrusio of the hip?*

Protrusio femoral head should be lateral to the ilioischial line but >3mm medial or >6mm medial in male vs female is abnormal. Most commonly this is idiopathic **OTTO's** pelvis 10:1 **female**, leading to arthritis in midlife. **Causes**: vascular, idiopathic / iatrogenic, trauma, autoimmune, metabolic, infective, inflammatory, neoplastic, congenital, dysplastic, endocrine, functional, genetic. **HIRST** classification <5mm, <10, <15mm protrusion (stages 1 to 3).

Q43. Management of protrusio?

If cartilage **open** surgical closure and **valgus** osteotomy. If **closed** just the osteotomy or THR if older (valgus osteotomy reduces JRF in medial side of joint which is the cause of progression).

Q44. How do you classify infection in relation of THR?

Fitzgerald:
- **Acute <3mth** superficial infection moves deep/infected haematoma
- **Delayed 3-24months** due to lower inoculation or lower virulence organism
- **Late >24month**: haematogenous seeding / change in host immunity

Q45. In your arthroplasty practice how would you prevent infection?

Pre-op: same day admission, separate trauma and elective units, shave in anesthetic room.
Peri op: Antibiotic loaded cement, systemic antibiotics, tissue handling, wash, reduce personnel in theatre, masks, suits, hair, double gloves, change gloves, drapes, ventilation and UV light.
Post op: recent UTI, abx catheter, patient factors (diabetic/ systemic disease control).

Q46. How do you decide if a THR is infected?

CRP>10 ESR >30 (Spangel, JBJS) 202 hips, all infections had at least one of these two raised, ESR sensitivity 82% specificity 86%, CRP sensitivity 96% specificity 92%.

Aspiration (Barrack, JBJS) on >200 hips sens 92% spec 97% false +ve 13%.

Frozen section >5PMN per mm^2, (**Mirra, CORR**) sensitivity 100% and specificity 95%.

Q47. How do you treat an infected revision case?

2 stage **Berend (CORR),** higher mortality, success up to 95%. Single stage revision, **Buchholdz (JBJS)** up to 91% success lower overall mortality.

Requirements for single stage revision success:
1) no sinus
2) no immunocompromise
3) good bone stock
4) 3-6months of abx post op
5) Known infecting organism's sensitivities

Q48. What are the indications for osteotomy of the hip in younger patients?

Indications: young, SUFE, Perthes, AVN, post # malunion, coxa vara /magna. **Contraindication**: stiff <90 flex, <15 deg abduction adduction, obesity, inflammation.

Varus femoral osteotomy: will shorten 1cm, pre-op abduction xr is required to ensure it's a feasible option, will move limb mechanical axis medially overloading medial side of the knee so need to translate medially to try to reduce this.

Valgus osteotomy: will need to do the opposite for same reasons and lengthens 2cm.

Intertrochanteric osteotomy: ideal for younger individuals with a history of femoral developmental anomalies such as coxa valga, coxa vara, Perthes disease, or slipped capital femoral epiphysis.

Valgus intertrochanteric osteotomy: most commonly performed for nonunion of a Pauwel class II or III femoral neck fracture.

Chapter 2: Adult Reconstruction Knee

Q1. ***Tell me about the lateral layers of the knee?***

Layer 1 Biceps, Iliotibial band, Nerve (*common peroneal nerve*).

Layer 2 Patella retinaculum, Patella femoral ligament.
Layer 3 (superficial): Fabello Fibula Ligament, LCL, Lateral geniculate artery.
Layer 3 (deep): Arcuate lig (fibula to oblique popliteal ligament), popliteo-fib lig, popliteus, capsule, coronary ligament.

Q2. ***Tell me the medial layers of the knee?***

Layer 1: Sartorius, Patella retinaculum, Gracilis, Tendinosis Saphenous nerve/vein
Layer 2: Membranosus, superficial MCL and posterior oblique lig → oblique popliteal lig
Layer 3: MCL (deep) and capsule

Q3. ***Give me the biomechanical strengths of these structures?***

1) MCL   **>4000N**
2) Quadrupled hamstring   **4000N**
3) Patella bone tendon   **2900N**
4) PCL   **2900N**
5) ACL   **2200N**
6) LCL   **750N**
7) MPFL   **110N**

Q4. ***What is the knee meniscus?***

- Cellular components are **fibrochondrocytes**
- Collagen type 1, 60% dry weight (overall 70% water)

- Collagen is arranged radially at the edge (shear) and circumferentially (centrally) to resist hoop stresses
- Blood supply is the medial and lateral inferior geniculate arteries

Q5. What is a discoid meniscus?

Bilateral in 25%, bow **tie sign** is the MRI finding, wide cartilage space seen on radiographs 11mm for the thick meniscus. **Watanabe** class I total, class II incomplete, III **wrisberg** variant – held only by meniscofemoral ligaments with deficient wrisberg-humphrey ligaments.

Q6. How does the meniscus tear?

Vertical (longitudinal) tear, radial (from the edge, best for repair), horizontal or degenerate. 0-5mm size good chance of repair with an appropriate injury with up to 85% healing rates.

Q7. What is its function?

- Stabilise
- Provide joint congruity
- Load sharing (50% in ext 85% in flex), total meniscectomy inc stress 234%
- Proprioception
- Articular lubrication / nutrition
- Shock absorption.

Q8. What other injuries are associated with damage to the ACL?

- >50% tear rate lateral meniscus.
- 20% MCL injury.
- **MRI shows lateral femoral condyle** and the **posterolateral aspect of the tibia** bone bruise in over 50% of patients (kissing lesions).

Q9. Is the injury relatively more common in males or females and why?

- 5x more common in **female** due to poor landing techniques in jump associated sports (volleyball), small notch/lig, hormones & valgus.

Q10. Tell me about tunnel placement for ACL surgery?

- **Femoral tunnel**: proper placement 1-2mm before post cortex of femur.
- **Tibial tunnel:** 10mm in front of the PCL anterior border. **Trajectory** of tunnels should be <75 deg from horizontal.

Q11. What happen when femoral tunnel placement isn't correct?

- Femoral tunnel - **anterior placement – think about anterior medial bundle of ACL (tight in flexion).** Leading to the knee that's **too tight in flexion** and **too loose in extension**. Usually caused by failure to clear **resident's ridge**. If placement too far back will lead to opposite – lax in flexion and tight in extension (*kind of what you want really – not really possible to do*).

Q12. What happen when tibia tunnel placement isn't correct?

- Tibial tunnel too anterior, knee will be tight in flexion (just like femoral tunnel) with impingement in extension. Posterior misplacement will cause impingement with the PCL.

Q13. You are a soft tissue knee surgeon so will you perform a double or single bundle ACL repair?

- **Classical single** vs **double** bundle ACL paper by **Ibraham & Adachi two RCT (JBJS)** showed that double bundle = slightly less translation possible post op but not significant clinical difference to the patients overall functional result.

Q14. Give me the anatomy and composition of the anterior and posterior cruciate ligaments?

- **Ligaments** are mainly collagen, 90% type I 10% type III
- **PCL** is approximately 38 mm in length and 13 mm diameter, **ACL** 33-11mm ACL

Q15. *Tibial eminence fracture classification?*

Myers and McKeever
1 undisplaced
2 partial hinged
3a ACL insertion injury
3b intercondylar notch injury
4 comminuted.

Q16. *Describe the different types of knee dislocation?*

Schenck knee dislocation classification I-IV

I ACL + collateral
II ACL & PCL
III ACL PCL + MCL or LCL (IIIL IIIM)
IV all

Q17. *Sequence of reconstruction after knee dislocation?*

- **MCL** can be conservative, hinge brace and get knee bending
- Reconstruct **posterior lateral corner** at 3wks
- **ACL PCL** at 6wks

Q18. *How would you rehabilitate an isolated PCL injury?*

Immobilize in extension – motion in prone position **not closed chain**.

Q19. Tell me about the LCL?

LCL (4mm diameter 66mm length). **Most anterior structure on the fibula head but originates behind the popliteus tendon on the femur.** Fibula head insertions from front to back 1) LCL 2) Popliteo fibula ligament 3) Biceps femoris. **Tightest against varus in 25 deg of flexion** (so tension a repair in this position). Becomes a restraint against external rotation in 50 deg flexion.

Q20. Technical considerations if performing a LCL reconstruction?

PLC reconstruction (varus lateral thrust gait) – lateral approach to knee between ITB and biceps. Bone patella bone if just LCL or fibula based reconstruction (Larson technique) figure of 8 with graft fixed to the femur or tendo-achilles graft fixed to isometric point on the femur epicondyle and one side to fibula head with bone tunnel and another passed through the tibia to re-create the popliteo fibula ligament.

Q21. Patella dislocations, what actually happens and surgical treatment options?

Patella dislocation – femoral insertion avulsion – soft tissues are the primary restraint until 20 deg flexion then bony structures take over and become total restraint at 40 deg of flexion, hence dislocation in the normal knee usually occurs before 40 deg flexion. Surgical options are for **reconstruction** or **repair** – recon with hamstring graft – femoral origin is at **shottle point** – just superior to blumenslats line in line with posterior cortical boarder on the lateral radiograph. Always assess the knee fully to decide best course of action as a Fulkerson osteotomy might be better if there is an increased Q angle or distailisation can be used for patella alta. **No bone procedures on patients with an open physis.**

Q22. What is lateral patella compression syndrome?

Improper tracking in the groove due to tight retinaculum, associated with miserable malalignment (femoral anteversion genu valgus ext rotation of tibia / pronated feet). Unable to evert the lateral edge of the patella and merchant view shows tilt. **Treatment**: strengthen the VMO or scopic lateral release (must have tilt and less than 1 quadrant patella glide). Another option is the Maquet (pure anterior translation of the tubercle 1cm), Elmslie Trillat or Fulkerson (not for any arthrosis).

Q23. Treatment options of osteochondral defects?

- **Osteochondral allograft transplant** – large defects.
- **Subchondral** 2.5mm **drilling** or **microfracture** 3-4holes per 1cm squared, best results from femoral lesions and if patient <40yrs.
- **Mosaicplasty (autologous osteoarticular transfer)** 2.5-8.5mm osteochondral plugs harvested from non wt bearing areas.
- **ACI (autologous chondrocyte injection)** – chondrocytes inj under a periosteal patch sewn to the defect (open). 12-5mm of cartilage harvested from the superior medial femoral condyle, 250,000 cells cultured to make 12million cells in 3-6wks then re-implanted and covered with periosteal flap from medial tibia, published by **Britberg** (**New Eng Journal of Medicine**).
- **MACI (matrix associated)** – delivery on a type I or type III collagen flap – avoid problems of the periosteal flap harvest, same culture etc.

Q24. What are plica in respect to the knee?

Asymptomatic synovial folds – 3 common found in the knee: **ligamentum mucosum** (in the notch), **suprapatellar plica** from medial to lateral in the suprapatellar space and the **medial plica** from the infrapatellar fat pad to the media side of the knee – causes symptoms by abrasion against medial femoral condyle. Can cause symptoms with resisted extension 'click' or pain.

Q25. Describe the important clinically issues associated with adolescent osteochondritis dissecans?

Usually the lateral side of the medial femoral condyle but can occur anywhere in the knee.

Worst prognosis in PFJ > Tibia > Femur. Fluid behind the lesion on MRI is also a poor prognostic indicator.

Classification **Clanton / Guhl** (same as Myers and Mckeever)

1 depressed fracture
2 fragment attached by bone 'hinge'
3 detached totally but insitu
4 displaced.

Pappas (prognostic indicators) increasing age at diagnosis equates to a worse prognosis.

Wilson test – pain with internal rotation of tibia during extension of the knee between 90-30 deg which improves with external rotation when you reach the pain point (like a meniscal provocation test rotating it away from the lesion helps). **Microfracture** lesions, or operate if impending physeal closure, signs of instability, longstanding lesions, expanding lesions, fix unstable lesion (>2cm in size tend to be unstable), chondral resurfacing for lesions greater than 2 by 2cm, bone pegs k wires or cannulated or Herbert headless screws to fix if required.

Q26. Tibial osteotomy for knee pain?

High tibial osteotomy:
- Varus/valg producing osteotomy gives a >85% good ten-year prognosis
- **Varus producing osteotomy:** for deformity less than 12 deg (or will result in very oblique joint line) – contraindicated in loss of medial meniscus or OA signs here as the osteotomy

will of course overload the medial compartment. Distal femoral osteotomy is better as the problem is in the femur **CORA** (deformity principles).

- **Valgus producing osteotomy:** closing wedge is better in that you can full wt bear, more stability and no bone graft requirement. Medial open wedge – maintains a posterior slope better and avoids deep peroneal nerve (advantages) the main problem is **patella baha** as your raising the joint line.

Q27. What type of patient might do well with an osteotomy rather than arthroplasty?

Ideal patient: <60yrs, has flexion 90 deg, -15 deg extension lag, single compartment OA, 15 deg varus max.

Q28. Contraindications to HTO?

1) loss of lateral joint space / subluxation >1cm
2) medial compartment bone loss >3mm
3) ligament instability
4) inflammatory arthritis

Q29. Surgical principles of HTO?

- Correct tib-femoral angle to at least or **over 8deg (Coventry** method, **JBJS).**
- **Overcorrection** to offload medial compartment.
- Thickness of wedge can be calculated via computer software.
- **HTO** for valgus knee so long as no more than 12 deg
- **>12deg valgus** = distal femoral osteotomy or the joint line will be sloped.

Q30. Types of TKR?

- **PCL retaining** - low conformity 'round on flat design' = inc roll back = **but** can edge load, lift off, slam down increasing contract stress and wear.
- **PCL stable** designs – confirming surfaces and cam achieve stability, but can 'cam jump' in high flexion knees.
- **Mobile bearing designs - advantages** less backside wear, will accommodate minor malrotation, **disadvantages** – dislocation / impingement of bearing

Q31. Should you resurface the patella?

- **Bernet (CORR), Campbell (JBJS**), both classical RCTs both found no difference but decision should be based on the implant and surgeon preference.

Q32. Sequence of release for 'tight knee' laterally and how do you deal with bone defects?

Lateral release – osteophytes → capsule → IT band (if extension tight) → Popliteus (if tight in flexion) → PCL → LCL & constrained implant. **Bone defects** <20% of cut surface and contained defect can bone graft it – uncontained defects 3mm or less can be undercut and use thicker poly, if >3mm use augmentation blocks or metaphyseal sleeves. If just keep cutting back you will change the joint line.

Q33. Prerequisites for a uni TKR?

1) Correctible varus.
2) Flexion to 110 deg.
3) ACL intact.
4) FFD less than 15 deg.
5) Intact contralateral compartment.
6) Non-inflammatory arthritis.

Q34. Do you know any developmental patella problems that may cause abnormal tracking?

Wiberg classification – patella shape – **type 1** medial and lateral facets are roughly equal (normal) **type 2** medial is larger **type 3** lateral is nonexistent really – all due to patella riding up on ridge during development causing dysplasia.

Q35. How do you define patella alta / baha respectively?

Patella alta/baha – Insall salvati index 1.2 to 0.8.

Q36. Describe the causes and treatment options for patella-femoral joint instability?

1) **Bone:** (dysplasia of patella or trochlea, condyle, alta.
2) **Soft tissue** MPFL or laxity.
3) **Malalignment**: femoral anteversion, torsion, TT TG distance, flat feet, genu valgum, Investigation should look for the cause: Patella tilt <10 deg, trochlear sulcus angle max 138 deg, anteversion of the hip 15 deg max, torsion of the tibia, TT TG distance <20mm, patella trochlear depth. Look for and treat the primary cause.

Q37. Tell me about patella-femoral joint replacements?

- Must have isolated arthritis PFJ or trochlear dysplasia
- **CONTRAINDICATED** in inflammatory arthritis / patella tracking problems
- **Ackroyd, (JBJS)** >300 lubinus implant - patient defined success rate as 80%, revision rate 96% survival at 5years although much worse on UK national joint registry

Q38. What are my treatment options for an arthritic knee?

- **Akmal (JBJS) - Hyaluronic acid injection** (incorporated into cartilage – improved chondrocyte density and reduced inflammation) may have role in patients who are active and over 60yrs and moderate arthritis.

- **Arthroscopic** synovectomy for rheumatoid, 83% improved outcome at 3yrs, valgus bracing and arthroscopic lavage **(Arron, JBJS),** 90% of patients with mild OA were improved with this at 2 years – but not for severe arthritis.
- **Arthroplasty** uni or total **(NJR).**
- **Constrained nonhinged prosthesis** varus valgus constraint for patients with a loose flexion gap or no MCL.
- **Constrained with hinge** for global ligament deficiency, polio, hyperextension instability, Charcot knee and MCL gone.

Q39. Types of instability after TKR?

- **Patello-femoral:** medialised femoral sulcus resulting in lateralisation of the patella.
- **Tibio-femoral**: flexion, global, varus or valgus.
- **Note: Patello-femoral maltracking** is most common reason revision 8-35% of cases. Elevated joint (baha) can cause tracking problems, lower joint (alta) will lead to flexion instability. **Joint Line** change of more than 8 mm reduces ROM, PFJ function/stability.

Q40. Tell me how you would manage an infected knee replacement?

- **TKR infection the scale of the problem:** 1% infection in primary 6% in revision.
- **Infection markers:** ESR 3 months to normalise CRP 3 weeks.
- **Bone scan** in all 3 phases suggests infection but remodelling during the first year makes this unreliable.
- **Infection < 30 days** – poly revision, synovectomy and wash can salvage **25%.**
- **Aspiration** WCC >1100 mm^3 = likely infection (>60% polymorphs).
- **Chronic Antibiotic Suppression**: success rate, symptoms control >25%.

- 2 stage revision proven by **Haleem (CORR)** 91% effective.

Q41. What is catastrophic wear in respect to TKR?

Premature failure of prosthetic implants due to excessive loading, macroscopic failure of PE, and mechanical loosening **not osteolysis /aseptic loosening**.

The main issues are
(1) PE thickness
(2) articular geometry - flat = point loading = high wear
(3) sagittal plane knee kinematics – sliding = bad
(4) PE sterilization techniques (oxidation etc.)
(5) PE manufacture creates sensitized stretched UHMWPE chains sensitive to oxidation and failure, can combat with compression molded components will reduce delamination and subsurface oxidation.

Q42. What's the ideal position for a knee arthrodesis?

5-8 degrees of valgus, 0-10 degrees of external rotation (to match the other foot), and 0-15 degrees of flexion.

Q43. Described the medial approach to the knee to fix a tibial plateau fracture?

Incision from ant tibia to post femur centered on middle medial joint line. Then incision on anterior boarder of sartorius. Under this is gracilis and below that semitendinosis – bend the knee and retract all 3 posteriorly to expose MCL and see the semimembranosus running under the MCL (in line of the pes) - can now go anterior to this into the joint or posterior to it into the posterior joint if you retract the medial head of gastrocnemius off the back or joint capsule / detach – **popliteal artery** is here so watch out. Medial geniculate artery is at superior boarder of the semi membranosus.

Q44. How about approaching a type II tibial plateau?

Anteriolateral approach to tibia L shaped curved incision across lateral joint and down at the patella tendon 3cm distal to the joint to begin with. Open joint and detach enough of lateral meniscus to perform the operation – then re attach. Work in a plane between periosteum and tib ant on the tibia.

Q45. How would you approach the posterior-lateral corner of the knee?

Incision between **biceps femoris** (sciatic) and **iliotibial band** (superior gluteal) ITB inserts into Gerdy's tubercle and biceps into fibula. Biceps (retracted backwards) will take common peroneal nerve away from the incision as it is separated from ITB (retracted forwards). Then you can enter the joint either side of LCL – behind by moving the lateral head of gastroc off and watch for vessels of **inferior lateral geniculate artery** in this area to be coagulated. Also, will find popliteus here moving through the joint capsule so its tendon is inside the knee. If the dissection to the repair posterior-lateral corner then extend the incision and isolate the **common peroneal nerve** and protect it (on back of biceps).

Q46. Describe the posterior surgical approach to the knee?

Incision down the biceps femoris laterally oblique across the joint line and then down the medial head of gastroc. At level of the fascia straight incision from bottom to top first identify the **small saphenous vein** at bottom of the incision and the **sural cutaneous nerve lateral** to it as you open the fascia. Find common peroneal and tibial nerves at top of the incision and dissect out to protect common peroneal. The fossa is boarded by semimembranosus medially and biceps laterally (find the nerve under biceps). Structures go artery vein nerve medial to lateral. Find the artery and vein next (deeper than the nerve) and may need to ligate some of the branches of the artery to mobilize (2 superior 2 inferior and one middle genicular artery). At this point can detach either head of gastroc to access the joint. The **common peroneal nerve** follows back of biceps around the lateral side of the knee and into **peroneus longus** muscle where it divides into superficial and deep.

Q47. What is iliotibial band friction syndrome?

Abrasion between the ITB and the lateral femoral condyle causes ITB friction syndrome. Running uphill and cycling, localized tenderness worse with knee flexed 30 degrees. The **Ober** test shows tightness in the ITB with the patient in a lateral decubitus position and the hip abducted and hyperextended. Nonoperative rehabilitation is the mainstay of treatment, but for refractory cases, surgical excision of an ellipse of the ITB can be effective.

Chapter 3: Statistics, Biomaterials & Physics

Q1. What different types of data exist?

Can be **Nominal** – not ranked (green red etc.) or **Ordinal** ranked (1st 2nd etc.)
Can be **qualitative** (nominal ordinal) or **quantitative** (numerical)

Q2. Tell me about variance, mean and standard deviation?

Variance is measure of spread, mean is measure of central tendency
Variance is the average of the squared differences about the mean
(x-mean) sq (added together) / n-1. **SD** is the sq root of the variance

Q3. What kinds of statistical errors can occur?

T1 error = found a difference but no difference exists (alpha should have been set lower eg 0.01 rather than 0.05) or too many tests used on the same sample (testing until you find something significant) or too many patients in the study 1000's rather than 100's.
T2 error = no diff found but there is one (beta) = not enough patients, low power to detect a difference.
T3 (sometimes called type 2 gamma) error = stats are perfect but authors conclusions are incorrect.

Q4. What criteria make a good screening test?

Wilson & Junger screening criteria = **IATROGENIC**

I = **important**
A = **accepted diagnostic** available
T = **treatment** available
R = can **recognize** early symptomatic stage
O = **opinion** on who to treat is agreed
G = **guaranteed** safe and sensitivity of the test
E = **examination** exists

N = **natural** history of condition known
I = **inexpensive** simple test
C = **cost** effective

Q5. *What's the difference between sensitivity and specificity?*

Sensitivity = ability of pick up all cases of disease = true pos / true pos + plus false negatives.
Specificity = ability to exclude disease = true neg / true neg + false positives.

Q6. *What levels of evidence can you describe in relation to a study paper?*

Oxford centre for evidence based medicine 2009
- **Level 1** = RCT, narrow confidence intervals or systematic review of RCT
- **Level 2** = RCT, lower follow up < 80% or cohort studies
- **Level 3** = case control or review of case control studies
- **Level 4** = poor quality case control, case series, low follow up cohort
- **Level 5** = expert opinion based on first principles

Q7. *Describe different types of lever in relation to human motion?*

1st class = fulcrum in centre, load and weight at opposite ends = atlanto occip joint
2nd class = weight in centre, force at one end and fulc at other = standing on toes
3rd class = force in centre and other two at either end = elbow

Q8. *Describe the various regions of the stress strain curve?*

- **Toe in region** for biological uncrimping collagen fibres leads to elastic region which follows hooks law.

- **Elastic region** - the material itself is insensitive to the rate of loading unless its viscoelastic, reaching the proportionality limit/ yield point.
- **Proportionality limit** – where elastic behaviour is no longer perfectly linear.
- **Plastic region** entered (at the **yield point**), further deformity is not recoverable, little stress = dramatic inc in strain, perfect plastic region then **strain hardening** = plastic deformation actually increased its resistance to further deformity = gradient of curve inc = cold working in metal alloys
- **Yield stress** – stress required to produce a certain amount of permanent deformation, in ortho the proportionality limit and elastic limit and yield stress are so close they are the same.
- **Necking** – cross sectional area of metal increases just before failure
- **Ultimate tensile stress** = the max before failure.
- **Fracture stress** = end of the graph.

Q9. What are the five types of force that can be applied to a material?

.

Five types of force - Bending, compression, tension, torsion, shear.

Q10. Tell me about stainless steel?

Stainless steel 316 – 63% iron, 18% chromium, 16% nickel, 3% molybdenum 0.03% carbon. Chromium and carbon increase corrosion resistance via oxide layer.

Q11. Tell me about titanium?

Titanium 64: 89% Titanium, Aluminum 6%, Vanadium 4%, as the alloy forms it forms an oxide layer by passivation good against corrosion.

Q12. Tell me about cobalt chrome?

Cobalt Chromium: 35% Nickel 34% Cobalt 20% Chromium 10% Molybdenum 0.02% Calcium.

Q13. What types of materials can be implanted surgically?

Polymers – Sutures, bearings, bio absorbable implants.
Metals – Joint replacements, screws, plates.
Ceramics – Bearings, dental implants.
Composite – Hydrocarbon joint replacements, heart valves.

Q14. What are ceramics?

Ceramics are compounds of metallic elements aluminum, zirconium silicone bound ironically or covalently to nonmetallic elements to form oxides. They have a granular microstructure. Implants are created from powered ceramics pressed into molds at high temperature.

Important properties:
- Insoluble
- Highly biocompatible (chemically inert at low energy state)
- Hard (high UTS)
- High elastic modulus and resistance to wear.
- Have no plastic deformation before failure (brittle).

Q15. What is a polymer, how are they created?

- **Polymer** = repeat sequence of monomer C-H with or without oxygen.
- Created via **addition polymerisation** - occurs by breaking double carbon bond with a free radicle. Or via creation of a water molecule which is **condensation polymerisation**.

- **UHMWP created via** condensation polymerisation, 5million repeating units, made through power casting low temp low pressure 4-6 bar.
- **Structure:** forms semi crystalline structure amorphous with random entanglement of chains good resistance to wear.
- **Sterilisation:** cannot be heated as melts at 130 deg, must be irradiated creating cross linking and increased strength if performed in an inert environment.

Q16. Tell me what's is in cement and how does it set?

- **Liquid** contains the 1) monomer 2) NN di methyl toluidine (accelerator) & 3) hydroquinone (inhibitor).
- **Powder** contains the 1) polymer 2) PMA a co-polymer 3) barium (radio opaque) and 4) benzyl peroxide (initiator)
- **Addition polymerisation reaction occurs when setting →** sandy →liquid →stringy →dough →exothermic reaction → hardening.

Q17. Femoral components have specific design features, tell me about composite beam vs taper fit designs?

- **Composite beam type stem (shape closed)** – anatomical design – creates a high shear/tensile stress and low compressive stress in relation to bone eg Charnley.
- **Taper fit (force closed)** – low shear/tensile, high compressive stress to bone – ability of cement-bone to undergo creep and stress relaxation makes this possible.

Q18. What is viscosity, what are synovial fluids made from and why is it special?

- **Viscosity** is the internal friction of a fluid.
- **Synovial fluid** is dialysate of plasma without clotting factors, cells or haemoglobin, hyaluronate, contains plasma proteins and metabolites.

- **Synovial fluid undergoes shear thinning** (as shear rate increases viscosity dec), this is derived from alignment of hyaluronate molecules.

Q19. What kinds of lubrication do you know within the knee joint?

- **Hydrodynamic** = high speed low load, during swing phase fluid film squeezed between two surfaces.
- **Elastohydrodynamic** = bearing surfaces change shape to trap fluid, increased surface area decreases shear rate and increased capacity of fluid film to carry load.
- **Microelastohydrodynamic** = asperities are deformed under high loads further increasing surface area spreading load.
- **Squeeze film** = as surfaces approach one another fluid is pressurised into the gap supporting load itself, occurs during heel strike.
- **Weeping** = local pressure generates weeping fluid out of cartilage to lubricate.
- **Boosted** = fluid pressurised into cartilage leaving behind hyaluronic acid protein complexes to lubricate surfaces in greater concentrations locally.
- **Boundary** = lubricin (glycoprotein) and phospholipid prevent direct contact.

Q20. What kinds of 'wear' can you describe?

Wear is the progressive loss of material from its bearing surface, can be **mechanical** or **chemical** (corrosion – unwanted dissolution of a material).

Mechanical wear can be:
- **Abrasive** (soft vs hard).
- **3rd body** abrasive.
- **Adhesive** (bonding b/w materials then damage as they move apart).
- **Fatigue** delamination due to fluctuating stresses.

Corrosive wear can be:

- **Galvanic:** electrically coupled active alloy becomes the anode = corrosion.
- **Crevice:** corrosion formation of a cavity acidic micro environment accelerates corrosion; low oxygen tension prevents formation a protective oxide layer.
- **Fretting:** synergy of crevice and wear, micro motion removes oxidised layer
- **Pitting**: similar to crevice within a 'pit'.
- **Stress**: corrosion increased/ accelerated with fatigued areas of the material.
- **Intergranular:** corrosion occurs at the grain boundary which is cathodic, alloys are more susceptible to this, intergranular leaching can occur
- **Inclusion:** corrosion occurs when cold welding introduces an impurity to the metal i.e. a screw driver leaving metal on a screw head.
- **Leaching**: like intergranular but actually in the grain not the boundary

Q21. What factors effect rate of poly wear?

- Surface roughness: damaged at time of implantation.
- Thickness: most poly requires at least 8mm (or early failure).
- Type of material
- Head size = greater sliding distance = greater volumetric wear
- Using metal back cups / tray = backside wear.
- 3rd body wear.
- Forces on joint (implanted correctly).
- Methods of manufacture (machining, impurity Ca-stearate and sterilisation).

Q22. What happens during aseptic loosening?

Activated macrophages respond to the release interleukins, cytokines, prostaglandins, and signaling from osteoblasts, absorb bone directly with hydrogen peroxide or stimulation of osteoclasts via IL1, 6, TNF alpha, prostaglandin E2, TGFB to directly absorb bone compromising implant stability, generating further particles 0.5-1 micrometers in size which active macrophages.

Overall osteolysis is determined by:
- Volume of wear debris.
- Total number of particles.
- Particle size & shape. **Size** in micrometres [0.02 ceramic / ceramic bearing] [0.05 to 0.5 metal-metal bearing] [0.5 to 100 metal-poly bearing].

Chapter 4: Basic science

Q1. What is osteonecrosis?

Osteonecrosis – death of cell population within bone. Usually effects 20-50yrs old's. Caused by interruption of circulation and doesn't directly affecting other organic or inorganic components. **Causes**: Idiopathic 40%, arterial disruption (fracture dislocation infection), thrombosis, nitrogen bubbles (Cassons), SLE (micro circulation), sickle, embolism, vasculitis, irradiation, fatty infiltration, steroid >30mg >30days, Gaucher's macrophages, alcohol, pancreatitis, hyperlipidemia, renal transplant, hematological malignancies, sepsis, inflammatory bowel disease.

Q2. Tell me how an xray is created?

Tungsten heated in a vacuum >2000 deg → thermionic emission produces electrons → move towards anode at 150 million meters per second, some hit nucleus of tungsten creating xrays, these are absorbed then hit the xray cassette (carbon fiber front, lead back and film in centre), phosphor crystals either side of the film (gadolinium) absorb xray and convert these to light which exposes film. Film is then processed by alkaline then, acid fixation.

Q3. How does ultrasound work?

Piezoelectric transducer produces the sound wave at 2-18MHz. Transducer detects the reflected sound wave and converts this into a digital image.

Q4. How is an MR image produced?

Patients tissue protons align with the magnet & wobble (**precession**), pulse (**radiofrequency**) causes re alignment to the pulse, this pulls precession **into phase** generating tiny magnetic fields, changes in these currents characterizes the tissue. Pulse stops and protons realign with the magnet causing a **longitudinal magnetization vector (electromagnetic signal)** this increase to maximum then falls creating the T1 signal = time this takes to recover to 63% of its max value. **De-phasing** then occurs as precession falls out of step, this causes **transverse magnetization** vector to fall from its max to 37% of it max value = T2 signal. MR converts these electrical signals into digital images depending on the density of protons in each and relative tissues.

Q5. What's a bone scan?

Tn^{99} isotope is injected (emits gamma radiation), isotope is formed from Molybdenum^{99} coupled with phosphate compounds to allow uptake into bone. Gamma camera contains crystals to absorb the radiation and convert into a digital image. At 1-2mins images are taken in the arterial flow hyper-perfusion phase, 3-5mins pooling phase, venous extracellular fluid volume and bone soft tissue hyperemia is seen and then at 4 hrs. images show skeletal activity (bone phase).

Q6. What is electrosurgery?

Electrosurgery alternating current. Monopolar involves a **high current small electrode** to generate heat at the tip and large surface area pad to return and avoid burns. Wave forms of **cut** and **coag** are different in % time of burst which is intermittent current. The system is **isolated** (with the plate) so cannot get a burn from 'grounding' through contact with metal areas of operating table. With bipolar the current passes between electrodes at the surgical site.

Q7. List the unique viscoelastic properties of biological materials?

- Creep
- Hysteresis
- Stress relaxation
- Shear thinning

Q8. What are tendons made from?

60% water, 80% type I collage (dry weight) some type XII (*t for tendon and t for twelve*). Can become more ***cartilage like*** in areas where they change direction / are subject to multidirectional forces other than tension (at bone tendon interface) – at this point have increased concentrations of type II collagen and proteoglycans. Cells are fibroblasts which become tenocytes (mature). Blood supply comes from synovial sheath, paratenon, muscle-tendon junction, periosteum, imbibition. **Ligaments** have lower water higher collagen content but are essentially very similar.

Q9. What is cartilage made from?

- 80% Water
- 10-15% Proteoglycans (fibromodulin, aggrecan, decorin)
- 10-20% Collagen (2, also 6 & 9 adheres cells + matrix, 10 = calcification)
- 1-5% Chondrocytes
- Others: cartilage oligometric protein, laminin, chondroadherin, chondronectin, anchorin, metalloproteinases and ions.

Q10. Tell me about the layers which compose cartilage?

In the **superficial zone**, the collagen fibers are parallel to the surface and are suited to the elastohydrodynamic form of joint lubrication. Low proteoglycan, high **water / collagen** concentration to resist shear and aid lubrication. **Transition + deep zones** contains fibers that have a larger diameter with less organization than in the superficial zone with a **high proteoglycan** concentration. **Tidemark** then **calcified zone** separates the deep zone of the articular cartilage from the subchondral bone anchors it with HA crystals, high type X collagen important for mineralization is found in this region.

Q11. What is a glycosaminoglycan made from?

Chondroitin and **keratin** sulphate form **glycosaminoglycans** when bound to a protein core like **hyaluronate** this forms a glycosaminoglycan **aggregate** = aggrecan, fibromodulin etc. Function is joint lubrication, reduce friction, shock absorption.

Q12. Can you describe the microstructure of muscle?

Muscle →fascicles made of fibers = elongated cells stuffed with→ **myofibrils**, made of **myofilaments** = the function unit of muscles made of actin and myosin, each fiber outer membrane invaginations are t tubules connecting to each sarcomere, to carry the action potential to muscle, surrounding each myofibril made up of myofilaments, is a membrane called sarcoplasmic reticulum – contains ca2+ which when released stimulates contraction.

Q13. Describe the structure?

- **Actin** 6 units surround 1 **myosin** component to make up a sarcomere
- 2 by 1 microns in diameter
- Hexagonal lattice, other structural proteins such as dystrophin maintain the structure

Q14. Function of bone?

1) reserve of calcium and phosphate
2) hematopoiesis
3) structure
4) movement

Q15. Types of bone?

Woven, immature, collagen random, no lamella, weaker more flexible, isotropic, rapid turnover, more cells. **Examples**: embryonic, neonate, pathological bone, callus, osteogenesis imperfecta, tumor bone.

Lamella, mature bone anisotropic character, parallel, collagen laid down by osteoblasts in sheets called lamella, cancellous (porous no specific osteons) or cortical, cement lines separate, mainly matrix with small number of osteocytes, in lacunae.

Cortical, 5-7 lamella (bone matrix) are arranged in columns of bone (containing osteocytes in lacunae) arranged into a **haversian system = or osteon**, each has a central neurovasc channel, each are encased within a cement line with Volkmas canals run perp to the axis carrying blood vessels.

Cancellous - 8x metabolic turnover, less brittle, less elastic, less dense, less strong

Q16. What is bone made from?

Bone, matrix 90% and cellular 10%, matrix inorganic comp = 60% = resist compressive mainly calcium and phosphate crystals, calcium hydroxyapatite (Ca10 PO4 6 (OH)2), brushite, strontium, lead, fluoride, 40% organic - resist tension forces, 90% of this is type 1 collagen, osteoblasts make this and hydroxylate it. Others – proteoglycans, osteonectin osteopontin osteocalcin = involved in mineralization, bone sialoprotein, bone morphogenic proteins, IL1 & 6 ILGF type 11- 12 collagen.

Q17. Describe bone metabolism?

7 dehydrocholesterol → in skin conv to **cholecalciferol** by sunlight = *active form of vit D3* also eaten. This is then hydroxylated in liver **25-hydroxycholecalciferol**, further hydroxylated at the proximal convoluted tubule of nephron to **1 – 25 dihydroxycholecalciferol**, in response to low Ca or phosphate or increased levels of PTH, - the opposite results in its conversion to inactive form of **24-25** form. PTH sec by chief cells of parathyroid in response to low Ca or phosphate or inhib by elevated levels of 1-25.1 -25 dihydroxycholecalciferol inc reabsorb in kidney of calcium and ex of phosphate in kidney and increased absorb of ca and phosphate in colon and stimulates osteoclasts.

Q18. What is the strain theory of fractures healing?

Perren's strain theory of fracture healing, depends on amount of strain at site, granulation tissue = strain up to 100%, fibrous tissue <17%, fibrocartilage <10%, lamella bone <2%. **Strain** at site depends on fracture gap, surface area, multi frag, type of fixation

Q19. Describe fracture healing?

Primary = **direct/haversian/osteonal** healing = compression and absolute stability – intolerant to strain at fracture site - new vessels grow across fracture gap, mesenchymal cells differentiate into osteoblasts laying down lamella bone in small gaps, woven bone large gaps – cutting cones follow behind containing osteoblasts/cytes creating osteons.

Secondary callous = relative stability defined as controlled motion b/w fractures surfaces under functional load, **first periosteal bony callous** = intramembranous ossification, osteo prog cells form bone without first forming cartilage – only at periphery so long as no stripping. **Second bridging callous** forms, enchondral ossification, cartilage precursor fibrocartilage, replaced by osteoid and woven bone.

Stage 1 **Hematoma** – fibrin clot, plts release of growth factors and cytokines, migration, prolif/diff **granulation tissue (type III collagen)**, neutrophils, fibroblasts, macrophages.

Stage 2 **Soft** callous – **fibrous tissue (type I collagen), cartilage and woven bone** = soft callous, intramemb ossification occurs, type 1 collagen by osteoblasts and matrix (osteoid) created by periosteal **osteoblasts**, hard callous (woven bone) not bridging. Enchondral fibrocartilaginous bridging occurs, cell diff into **chondroblasts** and **fibroblasts**, type 2 collagen and proteoglycan released into matrix which inhibit mineralization mainly cartilaginous chondroid **chondrocytes** then swell and apoptosis releasing $Ca2+$ and proteolytic enzymes which degrade proteoglycans and allows the fibrocartilaginous matrix to calcify.

Stage 3 **Hard** callous formation: soft callous is absorbed by **chondroclasts** – blood vessels invade bring osteoprogenitor cells, produce osteoid which mineralizes to form woven bone, mineralized woven bone, hard callous becomes united and pain free.

Stage 4 **Remodeling**– wolfs law remodeling depending on stress, coupled clastic activity and blastic activity.

Q20. How do bone grafts incorporate?

Cancellous: vascular ingrowth differentiation, chemotaxis, osteocytes that survive change to blasts, laying down new bone on the dead trabecular, **creeping substitution**, inc density on Xray, finally osteoblastic remodeling along lines of force then reduced density.

Cortical grafts are not incorporated. Enchondral bone formation occurs at the graft host junction and appositional bone formation – no remodeling occurs, allogenic grafts be destroyed by inflammatory response.

Vascular grafts – autogenous – incorporate same as for normal bone healing

Q21. *Types of bone graft?*

- **Osteogenic grafts**: contain live cells (only fresh grafts allo or autogenic).
- **Osteoconductive:** calcium phosphates.
- **Osteoinductive grafts:** such as fresh, freeze dried and fresh frozen allograft bone contain morphogenic proteins TGF-beta, FGF, PDGF.

Q22. *What is pseudohypoparathyroidism?*

PTH resistance at the end cell so **high** PTH. Can be **Albrights Hereditary Osteodystrophy**. Clinical **features** - skeletal defects, round, face, short, low IQ, brachydactyly, exostosis, effectively hypo parathyroid low Ca2+ high PO4, low vitD, rickets and osteomalacia.

Q23. *Describe the different types of rickets?*

Causes for rickets / osteomalacia:
- **Familial X linked dominant hyophosphataemic rickets** – due to renal unable to absorb phosphate, so low phosphate, labs normal but high ALP and low PO4, can be **called Vitamin D *resistant* rickets** *high dose vitamin D3 is the treatment.*
- **Nutritional Vit D *deficient* rickets** – malabsorption syndromes, infants, diet → low vit D levels so dec intestinal absorption of calcium, labs show low Ca low PO4 low Vit D, high PTH and high ALP in response, treatment is 5000IU vit D (calcitriol) daily will resolve the metabolic bone deformity.

- **Hereditary vitamin D _dependant_ rickets:**
  Type 1 deficient 25 hydroxylases so cannot produce active vitamin D
  Type 2 deficient receptor for 1-25, give high dose vitamin D plus elemental calcium

All result in renal osteodystrophy clinical features – browns tumors, looser zones, rugger jersey spine, wide growth plate, varus deformities, soft tissue calcifications, osteopenia, amyloid deposition

Q23. Tell me about osteoporosis treatment?

Bisphosphonates 50% fracture reduction over 3year period, Calcium and Vit D supplementation depending on age, elderly require 1500mg calcium 1000IU vit D / 24hrs

Q24 What do you know about Paget's?

Incidence: 3% in over 40s 10% in over 80yrs

Causes: Miners, family history in 30%, HLA DQW1

Pathology: **RANK** gene **OPG** genes abnormal, increased urinary hydroxyproline, ALP

Histology: Mosaic pattern of broad trabecular and disorganized cement lines and fibrosis

Radiographs: *Lytic* phase mainly at metaphysis
Active phase chaotic sclerosis and osteopenia combined
Burn out phase dense mosaic pattern of bone with little metabolic activity

Symptoms: Bone pain, OA, path fracture, deformity, nerve compression, conductive hearing loss, high output cardiac failure, spinal stenosis, gout, osteosarcoma

Q25. Tell me about BMP's?

BMP 1	Metalloproteinase that functions as enzyme for **collagen** types I, II, and III.
BMP 2	Osteoinductive factor that can induce **chondrogenic** change (mesenchyme).
BMP 3	**Inhibitor to other BMPs**
BMP 4	Overexpressed in fibro dysplasia ossificans progressive & HO (**mineralization**)
BMP 5	Plays a role in **osteoinduction**.
BMP 6 & 7	Located in hypertrophic cartilage and promotes **cartilage** maturation and eventual endochondral calcification.

Q26. What types of bone infection are there?

Cierney and Mader, 1990 anatomical classification:
Type 1 Medullary or endosteal infection
Type 2 Superficial infection
Type 3 Localized, well-marked infection with sequestration and cavity formation
Type 4 Diffuse osteomyelitis

Cierney Host types:
A – normal physiological response to the infection
B – impaired response either **L** = locally or **S** = systemically subtyped
C - treatment offers more compromising results to the patient than the disease process

Q27. Tell me about different types of antibiotics, how do they work?

Penicillin and cephalosporins	- Peptidoglycan cross-linkage
Glycopeptides (*vancomycin*)	- Inhibits cell wall production
Aminoglycosides (*gentamicin*)	- Inhibits 30S ribosome unit
Macrolides (*erythromycin*) & **Tetracycline**	- Inhibits 50S unit
Clindamycin & **Chloramphenicol**	- Inhibits 50S unit
Oxa-zolidin-ones (*linezolid*)	- Inhibits 50S unit

Rifamycins (*Rifampicin*)	- RNA synthesis
Fluoroquinolones (*Ciprofloxacin*)	- Inhibits DNA gyrase
Metronidazole	- Inhib DNA synthesis
Sulfonamides and trimethoprim	- Folic acid synthesis

Q28. *Which coagulation pathways do you know?*

Intrinsic Pathway factor 12 → 11 → 9 → 10
Extrinsic Pathway. Thromboplastin = TF + factor 7 → 10
Common Pathway. II (prothrombin to thrombin) → fibrinogen to fibrin

Q29. *Which cells are involved in bone turnover?*

Osteoblasts respond to PTH they sec ALP and type 1 collagen (bone matrix). Also, express **RANK** ligand which stimulates **osteoclasts** and **blasts**. **OPG** (produced by **osteoblasts**) bind RANKL and inhibits the whole process

Q30. *Layers of the growth plate?*

1) **Reserve zone** - store lipids proteoglycans and glycogen low oxygen
2) **Proliferative zone** - growth zone, stacking chondrocytes, increasing o2 and proteoglycan to inhibit calcification (achondroplasia effects this zone)
3) **Hypertrophic zone** - zones of **maturation, degeneration** and **provisional calcification**, chondrocytes swell with calcium, o2 levels decrease and cells undergo apoptosis – osteoblasts use cartilage scaffold and calcium to make bone. **Enchondromas** form in this zone, widens in **rickets**
4) **Metaphysis** cartilaginous bars replaced by lamellar bone

Q31. *Do you know any rules / laws of bone formation?*

- **Heuter Volkmas law** = compression over growth plate arrests growth
- **Delpechs law**   = tension over growth plate speeds up growth

Q32. *What is an EMG or a NCS electrophysiological test looking at?*

EMG:

Insertional activity in the muscle (as probe enters)
Activity at rest (should be silent)
Muscles **minimal contraction**
Interference pattern number, fire rates and recruitment pattern of motor units in that muscle (should be complete)

NCS:

Latency (measured in a few milliseconds)
Conduction velocity (40-45m/s)
Evoked response (biphasic)

Chronic axonal neuropathy   - all the above abnormal
Acute demyelinating   - conduction velocity 50% decreased
Neuropraxia   - **NCS** abnormal **proximal** to lesion
Axon/Neurotmesis   - **NCS** all abnormal
Ant horn disease/myopathy   - **EMG** abnormal

Chapter 5: Upper Limb Trauma

Q1. Where would you put ex-fix pins in the extremities?

- **Humerus** – pins go lat to medial in proximal half of the bone then front to back distally and finally laterally to medially at the elbow joint and condyles
- **Radius** – dorsally inserted pins in mid 1/3 and lateral pins in the distal 1/3 non-in proximal 1/3 as PIN not predictable – **ulnar** = anywhere posterior side
- **Pelvis** – supra acetabular pins go into ant inferior iliac spine b/w sartorius and TFL
- **Femur** – lateral pins but can go anterior in mid bone (this will be in the knee if ant distally)

Q2. Typical blood volumes for adults and children?

Estimate average blood volume 70ml/kg adult 80ml/kg, children (10yrs or less).

Q3. Immunization guidelines?

HPA guidelines: If fully immunized no need for vaccine if patient is high risk or wound high risk can give tetanus immunoglobulin (250IU for adult's x 2 if greater than 12hrs since injury), if immunization incomplete or unknown need to complete course – give vaccine and then 5 further doses – also require the immunoglobulin (<5yrs 75IU 5-10yrs 125IU).

Q4. What are the indications for damage control orthopaedics vs early total care?

- **ISS** score >40
- **ISS >20** with **chest injury**

- **Lactate >2.5mmol/l or IL6 >5mcg/l** = red flag for ETC, ideal lactate <2
- Multi injury pelvis abdo and shock
- Bilateral femoral fractures
- Hypothermic patients <35 deg and head injury.
- Acute inflammatory window is 2-5 days only life-threatening injuries should be treated in this time period eg unreduced dislocations, vascular injury, spine, compartment syndrome, open fractures, long bone fractures.

Q5. How do you calculate ISS?

Sum of squared results of the three biggest scores from the most severely injured body regions (nine regions) = max score of 75. Minor, moderate, serious, severe, critical, not compatible with life (1-6).

Q6. What kinds of necrotizing fasciitis are there?

Type 1 = **non-group A step**, anaerobes, enterobacteria, clostridia and synergic organism 90% of cases are type 1, usually type B hosts (unhealthy individuals)
Type 2 (healthy people) mono microbial organisms group A strep 5% of patients
Type 3 marine vibrio vulinficus (-ve rod)
Type 4 MRSA, the overall mortality for all causes is above 30%.

Q7. BAPRAS & BOA open fracture guidelines?

Cefuroxime 1.5g or 1.2g co-amoxiclav or clindamycin 600mg 6hrly if allergic. Plus, further dose at debridement and gentamycin 1.5mg/kg dose continued at this dose x3 daily for 72hr at least or until definitive wound closure. Wound cover 3-7days.

Q8. What is a MESS score in relation to extremity trauma?

Amputation score of 7 or more = amputate, '*MESS*' score –
Johannson 1990 (J. Trauma)

Energy	Simple	1
	Medium (open#)	2
	High (crush)	3
	Contamination	4
Shock	**BP < 90** (transient)	1
	Always <90	2
Age	30-50	1
	50+	2
Ischemia	Pulse reduced	1
	Paresthesia, < CRT	2
	Cool insensate dusky	3 (double if >6hr)

Q9. Draw the brachial plexus?

ROOTS: find between scalene anterior and middle
- Dorsal scapular nerve (C5)
- Branch to phrenic nerve (C4-5)
- Long thoracic nerve (C5-6-7)
- First intercostals nerve (C5)

TRUNKS: find in the posterior triangle (upper middle and lower)
- Suprascapular nerve(C5-6)
- Nerve to subclavius (C5-6)

DIVISIONS: find at the clavicle
- Anterior divisions of upper and middle trunk → lateral cord
- Anterior division from the lower trunk → medial cord
- Posterior divisions become → posterior cord

CORDS: find in the axilla around the axillary artery

Q10. Brachial plexus injury classification?

1) **Complete** (75%) or **incomplete**
2) **Supraclavicular** or **infraclavicular** (DSN, SS, LTN = if ok = **infra**)
3) Eponymous **Kumpke** (C8 T1) in 3% or **Erb** palsy (C5-6) in 20%
4) Mechanism, eg **high** energy / **low**
6) **Pre** or **post** ganglionic – if SNAP preserved on NCS then pre-ganglionic lesion
7) Cause – iatrogenic (anesthetic), radiation, obstetric

Q11. *What is a floating shoulder?*

Injury to the ring:
1) glenoid fossa
2) coracoid process
3) coracoclavicular ligaments
4) distal clavicle
5) acromioclavicular joint
6) acromial process.

Traumatic disruption of **2 or more** components requires surgical treatment because the shoulder will collapse anteriorly, inferiorly, and medially **Goss (JBJS)**

Q12. *What is a flail shoulder?*

Scapulothoracic dissociation: disruption of the scapula from the chest wall. This injury often presents with a flail, pulseless, swollen extremity after high-energy trauma and is life-threatening. A lateral shift of the scapula is seen on chest radiographs, and associated injuries include avulsion of the subclavian, axillary, and brachial arteries (>80%) and/or complete brachial plexopathy (>80%).

Q13. *Classification of AC joint injuries (Rockwood)?*

   (I) Sprain of AC

(II) AC joint disrupted, sprain of CC ligaments Less than 50% shift

(III) AC and CC ligaments gone deltoid and trapezius detached from clavicle AC joint dislocated with clavicle up to 100% displaced

(IV) AC and CC ligaments disrupted as above but backwards displacement

(V) As above up +100% superior displaced

(VI) Under coracoid.

Evidence: **Spencer (CORR)** type III injury or less = conservative management.

Q14. Classification of distal clavicle injury (Neer)?

Type 1 between ligaments / distal to ligaments remains undisplaced

Type 2a 56% nonunion fracture is medial to ligaments so big displacements

Type 2b between ligaments but with ruptured conoid (big displacement) or both ruptured and fracture is lateral to them v big displacement so high nonunion 45%, **type 3** intra-articular

Type 4 physeal

Type 5 comminuted – may operate for this as well as non-union

Hill (JBJS) & Canadian orthopaedic society found the 2cm rule - consider ORIF.

Q15. Classification of scapula injury?

Zdravkovic + Damholt
Type 1 = body
Type 2 = coracoid and acromion # ORIF if possible,
Type 3 = neck and glenoid #s = ORIF if large unstable

Indications for surgery scapular neck Goss (JSES) >40 deg or 1cm displacement

Q16. Indications for surgery to a glenoid fracture?

Ideberg, ORIF if:
>5mm step / gap
* >25% surface involved#
* scapula neck fracture with Goss criteria
* open fractures
* loss of cuff function
* poly trauma mobility issues

I	Anterior / posterior avulsion fractures (a or b)
II	Transverse/oblique fracture # exits inferior
III	# exits upper 1/3 of glenoid inv coracoid
IV	Horizontal glenoid# through body
V	Combination of II+IV (a), III+IV (b), II+III+IV (c)
VI	Comminution

Q17. Tell me about humerus fractures?

Neer classification ("part" is defined as displacement of more than 1cm **or** angulation of 45 degrees) so an impaction fracture can still be a 1-part fracture.

- **Humeral shaft fracture** 90% healing over 3months.
- **Kleinerman(JBJS)** publication demonstrated 20 deg AP and 30 deg varus and 3cm shortening is well tolerated.
- **Eikholm (JOT)** with radial nerve palsy no difference in recovery if it is presenting feature with ORIF or conservative treatment.
- **Radial nerve exploration for palsies associated with open fractures** is only indication that is not associated with conflicting data.

Q18. Describe capitellar fractures?

Technique tip: bury headless screw from ant to posterior as blood supply comes from the back if ORIF is performed.

Brian and Morrey classification:
Type 1 large capitellar # fix if >2mm displaced or 3wk cast.
Type 2 articular surface seared off – leave if undisplaced or excise if displaced.
Type 3 comminuted – leave or excise,
Type 4 (**McKee** addition) shear fracture including the trochlear in a type 1 – ORIF if displaced 2mm.

Q19. Describe some condylar fractures of the elbow?

Milch classification:
Type 1 smaller overall - lateral trochlear ridge intact – not part of the fracture,
Type 2 larger fragment lateral trochlear ridge is part of the fracture

Treatment – point thumb towards the fracture (put ligament attachment on stretch to reduce fragment to its anatomical position)

Epicondylar fracture described by Granger – immobilize for 2 wk or excise

Q20. Describe elbow coronoid fractures?

Regan and Morrey classification:
operate for instability when present

Type I	Tip fracture
Type II	Fracture of 50% or less
Type III	>50% of coronoid

Q21. Describe other elbow fractures?

Colton (olecranon) A= avulsion B= transverse/oblique C= comminuted D= dislocation

Mason radial head fractures:

Type I	Nondisplaced
Type II	Partial articular with displacement (ORIF if block to ROM)
Type III	Comminuted involving whole head (can ORIF if 2 distinct fragments of the head but if more, then excise or replace)
Type IV	As above ligamentous injury or other fracture – must have radial head implant

Q22.   What type of Monteggia fractures do you know?

Bado classification

Type 1	Anterior radial head dislocation
Type 2	Posterior radial head dislocation
Type 3	Lateral radial head dislocation
Type 4	Anterior radial head dislocation and proximal third radius #

Q23.   Talk about elbow fractures in children?

- Medial condyle fracture can accept up to 15mm displacement (*controversial*)
- Lateral condyle can accept 5mm max (*controversial*)
- **Humerus** can accept 45 deg and 50% apposition max
- **Gartland Type III supracondylar** fracture – **Leet (JPO)** >150 patients found no problems with 21-hour delay.
- Late presenting radial head dislocation (4wks) will need open reduction and may need triceps strips to reconstruct the annular ligament to maintain and reduction.

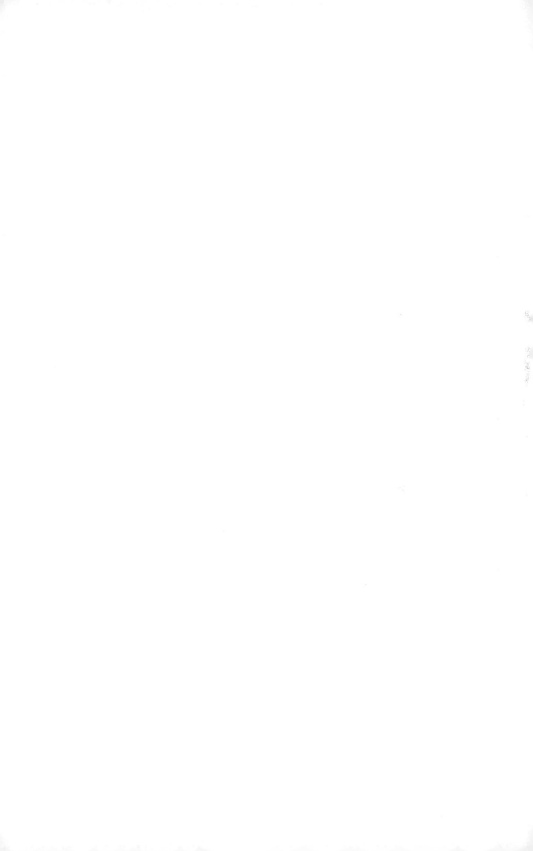

Chapter 6: Lower Limb Trauma

Q1. When should we treat an acetabular fracture non-operatively?

Matta criteria (CORR):
- Minimal displacement <2mm
- Draw roof arc angles should be >45 deg on AP oblique and lat – if # outside this area = relative stability good for non-operative management (**Matta, CORR)**
- >10mm from wt bearing dome = good sign for conservative treatment
- Posterior wall fracture <20% (as not unstable)

Good indications to operate:
- Opposite of the above
- Irreducible fracture dislocation or fragment in joint

Q2. Describe acetabular fractures?

Letournal classification:

Elemental
- Post wall, post column, ant column, anterior wall, transverse

Associated
- Post and anterior column injury
- **Next 4: are all Y or T shape** configurations, PP, TP, T, APH.
- **PP** = post column-post wall (t shape with line going down +back to ischium)
- **TP** = transverse with post wall (Y shape)
- **T** = t shape - transverse with fracture line going down to complete the T
- **APH** = anterior column with posterior hemi transverse; a posterior transverse type splitting into Y configuration at centre of acetabulum one limb going up anterior column and the other into pubis

Q3. Describe pelvic ring fractures?

ABC OTA / Tile classification:

A1 Avulsion not inv ring
A2 Inv ring minimal displacement
A3 Dennis zone III fracture through the sacrum

B1 Open book external rotation injury
B2 Lateral compression injury (one side internally rotates) internal rotation injury
B2-1 Ant ring through same side rami
B2-2 Through contralateral rami
B3 Bilateral (one side internally rotated one side externally rotated).

C Rotationally and vertically unstable
C1-1 Iliac wing up
C1-2 SI joint up
C1-3 Through sacrum and hemi pelvis up
C2 (bilateral hemi pelvis injury) one side is type B one side is a type C and
C3 A type C on both side of the pelvis.

Young and Burgess (Lateral compression) = *injury moves from one side to other*

LC 1 Transverse rami / sacral compression **(granny fracture)**
LC 2 Rami and iliac wing # or SI (internal rotation of one hemi pelvis)
LC 3 Same as type 2 but with contralateral external rotation caused by bilateral SI injury

Young and Burgess (AP compression) – *injury moves from front to back*

AP 1 Symphysis <2.5cm or vertical rami and anterior SI ligament **(non-operative)**
AP 2 **(ORIF or exfix)** – symphysis >2.5cm and SI joint and ligaments gone

AP 3 As above but posterior SI ligaments now gone, a true open book injury (**ORIF**)

Young and Burgess: Malgaigne (vertical shear) Anterior and posterior vertical displacement Acute external fixation/anterior ORIF if concurrent laparotomy; posterior SI ORIF (SI screws, anterior SI plate).

Q4. Femoral head fracture classification?

Pipkin:

Type I	Exits below fovea
Type II	Above it
Type III	Associated with femoral neck fracture (highest AVN)
Type IV	Associated with acetabular fracture

Q5. When and how would you fix a femoral neck fracture in a 40-year-old?

- **Conflicting evidence to prevent AVN** – pre or post 24hrs fixation (no difference)
- V pattern 3 screw technique by **Oakie (CORR)** reduced risk of subtrochanteric #
- Good spread of screws **Parker (JBJS)** = mechanically stronger, less risk non-union
- DHS for basocervical fractures gives stronger construct but higher risk of AVN

Q6. Where should DHS screw be targeted and how does the construct work?

- **Dead centre** or **post inf - Bawngardner (JBJS)** described the tip apex
- DHS acts as a tension band

Q7. What are the UK Nice guidelines 'Management of Hip Fractures in Adults'

1. Treat for next day / day of admission surgery
2. Reverse co-morbidity before surgery
3. Use implants / techniques to allow early wt bearing surgical techniques
4. Sliding hip screws not nails unless transverse / reverse oblique fracture
5. THR if patients not cognitively impaired and can walk with a stick outdoors or better
6. Anterior-lateral approaches
7. Cemented implants
8. Orthogeriatric input
9. Daily physio
10. Integrated NOF# pathway in the trust
11. Don't use NSAIDs

Q8. What is the National hip fracture database

- Over 180+ eligible hospitals UK collecting data
- Set up in 2007 – incorporation of BOA British Geriatric Soc and NICE guidelines
- Best practice tariff – to bench mark standards against these guidelines (6 steps):

1. admit within four hours
2. surgery within 48 hours
3. pressure ulcers
4. pre-op orthogeriatrician
5. bone protection medication
6. falls assessment prior to discharge

Q9. How would you manage femoral shaft fractures in children?

AAOS guidelines:
- <6yrs use spica or traction (<2yrs = spica)
- Accept 10deg angulation / 2cm short

- 6-13yrs use flexible nails / plate / traction 1cm overgrowth may occur in patients
- 14yrs+ as per adults

Q10. When could a retrograde femoral nailing be useful?

- If there is same side knee injury or a need to wash out the knee
- If bilateral injury then no need to re position patients (poly trauma)
- Preserves a pelvic approach (poly trauma)

Q11. Knee dislocations?

Classification can be directional (position of the tibia):
- **Anterior** 50% hyperextension intimal tears of the popliteal artery
- **Posterior** 25% axially loaded flexed knee, highest rate of complete vascular injury
- **Lateral** 13% valgus force highest rate of peroneal nerve injury
- **Medial**
- **Rotational** usually posterior lateral and pure rotational

Shencke classification (based on number of structures injured)
One ligament, two, three, four etc. Five is with a fracture.

Q12. Lauge-Hansen classification?

Based on the **foot's position** (first word of classification) and **motion** (talus) relative to the leg (second word of classification)

Supination-Adduction
Stage 1 Low transverse fracture of lateral malleolus or lateral collateral ligaments
Stage 2 Oblique fracture of the medial malleolus

Supination-External *(goes clockwise around the right ankle from lateral->medial)*
Stage 1 Rupture of the anterior inferior tibiofibular ligament
Stage 2 Oblique or spiral fracture of the lateral malleolus
Stage 3 Rupture of the post–tibiofibular lig or fracture of the posterior malleolus
Stage 4 Transverse (sometimes oblique) fracture of the medial malleolus

Pronation-Abduction *(straight across again but injury to the middle this time)*
Stage 1 Rupture of the deltoid ligament or transverse fracture of the medial side
Stage 2 Rupture of the anterior+posterior inferior tib-fib ligaments or bony avul
Stage 3 Oblique fracture of the **fibula at the level of the syndesmosis**.

Pronation external rotation *(rotation from medial to lateral clockwise anterior)*
Stage 1 Rupture of the deltoid ligament or transverse fracture of the medial side
Stage 2 Rupture of the anterior inferior tib fib ligaments or bony avulsion
Stage 3 Spiral/oblique fracture of the **fibula above the level of the syndesmosis**
Stage 4 Rupture of the posterior inferior tib fib ligament or fracture post malleolus

Q13. *Important angles for calcaneus fractures?*

- **Bohler** angle (25 to 40 degrees)
- Angle of **Gissane** (120 to 145 degrees)
- **Calcaneus fractures** 9 factors associated with poor outcomes: >50yrs, obesity, work comp (FFF – fat fifty and financial gain) MMM (manual workers, men, multi trauma), smoking, bilateral, vascular problems (**Buckley**)

Q14. Navicular fracture classification?

Sangerozan:

Type I	Fractures are in the coronal plane (splits it into dorsal - plantar fragment)
Type II	Classic fracture on the AP
Type III	Navicular body +comminuted → AVN → forefoot abduction

Chapter 7: Foot & Ankle

Q1. *How can you classify diabetic ulcers?*

Wagner classification:
0 Ulcers have intact skin (bony deformities may be present)
1 Localized superficial ulcer
2 Deep ulcer to tendon, bone, ligament, or joint
3 Deep abscess or osteomyelitis
4 Gangrene of toes or forefoot
5 Gangrene of entire foot

Q2. *How can we classify Charcot?*

Eichenholtz stages (mnemonic **dis-co resolution**)
I	(**dissolution**) Demineralization of regional bone, periarticular fragmentation
II	(**coalescence**) Absorption of osseous debris new bone formation increased stability
III	(**resolution**) Smoothing of edges of large fragments of bone, osseous ankyloses

Brodsky types:
1	TMT
2	Peri talus
3a	Ankle
3b	Post calcaneus
4	Multi sites
5	Forefoot

Q3. *Ankle replacement or fusion?*

- **Saltzman (FAI) replacements** gives superior pain relief at 2yrs
- Replacement vs fusion, **best** in **bilateral, Rh, multi joint**

- **Gougoulias (CORR)** systematic review about 90% 5 yrs survival for TAR

Q4. Which nerves does the medial plantar nerve innervate?

- 4 muscles, lumbricals (3rd & 2nd toes), abductor hallucis, FHB FDB
- Lateral planar nerve innervates the rest

Q5. Describe the 4 layers of the foot?

3-4-3-4 (muscles in each layer)

1st layer are the two muscles either side of the calcaneus **Abductor hallucis** and **abductor digiti** minimi then fill the gap with lots of tendons = **flexor digitorum brevis (both sides of middle phalanx)**.

2nd layer two extrinsic tendons **FHL FDL**, two special muscles **quadratus plantae** (both side of calcaneus to the lateral side of FDL and **lumbricals** (from FDL to ext hood act like hand lumbricals from medial sides of 2-5th MT)

3rd layer FHB (from cuboid & lat cuneiform into both side of base of proximal phalanx inserted into both sesamoids), **adductor hallucis** (has oblique head 2-4MT and transverse head from plantar plate of 3-5th MTPJs inserted into lateral side of proximal phalanx) and flexor **digiti minimi brevis** (base of 5th MT to base of proximal phalanx)

4th layer interossei plantar (MT to proximal phalanx and EDL) and **dorsal** (to the EDL and side of proximal phalanx), two extrinsic tendons – **tibialis post** and **peroneus longus**.

Q6. Tibialis posterior dysfunction flatfoot progression?

Classification Johnson, Strom & Myerson's addition:

Stage 1: tenosynovitis – no deformity
Stage 2a: deformity - normal forefoot but flexible valgus hindfoot
Stage 2b: abnormal hind and forefoot deformity **30% talar uncoverage**
Stage 3: fixed deformity
Stage 4: involving ankle deformity

Q7. Angles on the foot radiograph to define a flatfoot?

	Normal
Talo-navicular coverage angle	<7deg
Meary's	<5deg
Calcaneal pitch	18-20deg
Talocalcaneal angle	25-45deg
Kite ankle	15-30deg

Q8. Tell me how you would manage a TA rupture?

- 18 per 100,000, early wt bearing with protected ROM is equal to cast and non wt bearing in non-op treated ruptures **Willits (JBJS)** but need serial US for initial period with up to 20% failure (gap >1cm) and conversion to surgery
- <3 weeks can repair end to end, longer then may require additional procedures
- <4cm gap may require V-Y
- >4cm defect will require FHL transfer / augmentation
- **Classic paper = Nistor (JBJS)** +100 patient's TA rupture 4% vs 8% re rupture rates (surgery vs cons)

Q9. Berndt and Harty classic Xray classification of OCD?

Stage 1	Small subchondral depression
Stage 2	Partial detachment
Stage 3	Complete detachment
Stage 4	Complete detachment and displaced.

Treatment: intact surface = retrograde drill / graft from below or remove fragment and drill base, ORIF vs osteochondral grafting.

Q10. What is tarsal tunnel syndrome?

Compressive neuropathy of tibial nerve, can be:
INTRINSIC tenosynovitis, osteophyte, lipoma, tumor, fibrosis, ganglion
EXTRINSIC shoes, trauma, deformity, scaring, systemic inflammatory, oedema.

Q11. Describe the blood supply to the foot?

<u>**DP** artery divides into:</u>
> **deep plantar artery** to the sole of the foot
> **first dorsal metatarsal artery** (at risk - bunion surgery)
> **lateral tarsal artery** supply talus and join **peroneal** into **artery tarsal sinus**

<u>**Posterior tibial artery** divides deep to the abd hallucis muscle into:</u>
> **artery of the tarsal canal** primary blood supply to talus
> **calcaneal and deltoid branches** (around medial malleolus)
> **lateral plantar** deep to flexor digitorum brevis muscles
> **medial plantar** to form the deep plantar arch in the fourth layer of the foot

Q12. How would you diagnose and treat ankle instability?

Symptoms plus 5 deg difference in talar tilt on xrays or 10 deg absolute tilt or 5mm anterior draw difference or absolute 10mm anterior draw suggests instability.

Brostrom procedure - detach ATFL mid substance and double breast onto suture anchors and then **Gould modification** reinforcing the ATFL repair with overlap of the nearby lateral talocalcaneal ligament plus inferior <u>extensor ankle retinaculum</u>.

Q13. Explain gait?

- **Stance Phase**. 62% of the gait cycle, double-limb support 12% of the cycle,
- **Swing Phase**. 38% of the cycle (initial-mid-terminal swing 3 phases).

Initial contact
Loading response
Mid stance
Terminal stance
Pre-swing

I Like My Tea Pre-Sweetened

- **Step** is the distance between initial swing and initial contact of the same limb
- **Stride** is initial contact to initial contact of the same limb
- **Velocity** is a function of **cadence** (steps per minute) and stride length

Q14. Anatomy of the shoe?

1. Toe box (anterior portion of a shoe's upper),
2. Quarter (posterior aspect of a shoe's upper),
3. Counter (area at rear of shoe that encases heel and holds it in position),
4. Vamp (anterior aspect of shoe's upper)
5. Outsole (part of shoe that contacts ground) – heel, sole, shank, toe spring.

Q15. What are inlays made from?

- **Accommodative orthoses** are often made of **Plastazote**- provide minimal biomechanical alteration (life span of 2 to 6 months)

- **Functional orthoses**: semirigid/rigid - cross-link polyethylene foam/ rubber

Q16. *What types of theatre are there?*

* **Plenum**   20 air changes /hr- at the centre up to 300 cfu/m3
* **Laminar**   300 air changes /hr - at the centre <10 cfu/m3

Chapter 8: Hand & Microsurgery

Q1. How can you treat a Swan neck deformity?

Nalebuff (PIPJ tightness dictates treatment):

Mobile joints	**Splinting or lat band trans volar to prevent hyperextension**
Intrinsic tightness	**Intrinsic release & FDS advancement**
Globally tight / OA	**Fusion or replacement**

- Same for a **boutonniere** 1. Splint 2. Repair 3. Reconstruct 4. Replace 5. Fuse

Q2. Can you demonstrate a Kirk Watson test?

Thumb volar tubercle fingers dorsal (put patients elbow on table hand up and palm to you), radial deviated hand with your other hand (scaphoid will flex) then ulnar deviate (scaphoid with extend). On scaphoid flexion your thumb pressure will sublux the scaphoid dorsally on the radius (indicates rupture of the SL ligament – dorsally). Positive result is a 'click' or 'pain' but can be 'normal in 1/3 of patients.

Ballotment test (Reagan) – is the same for triquetrum and lunate.

Q3. Do you know any tests of the DRUJ / ECU?

- **Piano key** – hold distal DRUJ then press ulnar volar with other hand
- **Dimple sign** – traction to wrist and press ulnar DRUJ **dimple** suggest subluxation
- **ECU sublux** – ulnar deviate and extend – may displace the tendon / sublux

Q4. What is a Bennett's fracture?

Occurs when a flexed metacarpal is axially loaded. **Bennett fragment** consists of the volar portion of the metacarpal base that remains attached to the anterior oblique ligament. Adductor pollicis displaces the metacarpal head displaced into palm and APL causes the rotational deformity.

Q5. How would you reduce a Bennett's fracture?

1. Traction
2. Extension
3. Pronation
4. Abduction (thumbs up position)

* Less than 30 degree / 4mm short can be accepted

Q6. Indications for scaphoid fixation?

- Unstable fractures (includes displacement >1mm)
- Intra scaphoid angle >35deg
- Oblique waist (relatively unstable) for high demand patient
- If operating anyway for other reasons
- SL **angle greater than 60 degrees** (normal is up to 60 degrees) = instability sign

Q7. Surgical options for scaphoid fixation in a nonunion?

- Vascularised bone graft 1-2intercompartmental retinacular artery for necrosis proximal pole.
- The inlay (Russe) technique is best used in cases with minimal deformity
- **Humpback deformity** requires an opening-wedge interposition (**Fisk) graft** to restore scaphoid length and angulation with compression screw

Q8. Scaphoid fracture classification?

Herbert classification

A	Stable	incomplete waist A1 or tubercle A2 (distal)
B	Unstable	complete waist B1 B2 B3 distal mid proximal pole, B4 #dislocation
C	Delayed union	
D	Nonunion D1 fibrous (stable) D2 displaced (unstable)	

Q9. Wrist fracture classification?

Frykman (even numbers the same with ulnar styloid fracture)

I	Extra articular
III	Into joint
V	Into radio ulnar joint
VII	Enters both radiocarpal and DRUJ

Q10. What are the intrinsic ligaments of the finger?

- **Sagittal bands**
- **Conjoined lateral bands** – lumbricals, indicis, dorsal interossei
- **Oblique retinacular ligament** from lat volar aspect of prox phalanx inserts on lat terminal ext tendon
- **Triangular** ligament
- **Transverse band** origin from flex tend sheath of PIPJ ins into lat boarder of **conjoined lat bands** there to stabilise lateral bands and stop them displacing dorsally in extension

Q11. Intrinsic minus hand?

Deformity: MCP hyperextension, DIP PIP flexion (claw hand)

Causes: Ulnar tunnel, cubital tunnel, Volkmas, leprosy, failure to splint in neutral crush, CMT, compartment syndromes.

Management: Bring MCPJ out of hyper ext to see if you have passive ROM to see what needs to be done. Surgery for contracture release – passive tenodesis or tendon transfers to correct the deformity to prevent MCPJ hyperextension.

Q12. Intrinsic plus hand?

Deformity: DIP PIP extended and MCP is flexed (extrinsic vs intrinsic)

Causes: Trauma, vascular, compartment, Rh, neuro, CP, an imbalance. Test for intrinsic tightness

Surgery: Stretching or muscle slide soft tissue balance procedures

Q13. Wrist instability, what types do you know?

Carpal instability dissociative
- Volar intercalated segmental instability (VISI)
  Scapho lunate angle < 30 deg, strong positive capito lunate and radio lunate angle >30

Carpal instability dissociative
- Dorsal intercalated segmental instability (DISI)
  Scapho lunate angle >60 deg, capito lunate and radio lunate normal angles

Carpal instability non-dissociative
- Mid / ulno / radiocarpal = disruption of extrinsic ligaments

Carpal instability complex
- Scapho lunate – capito lunate – luno triquetral ligament – to radio lunate disruption clockwise injury described as the …

Mayfield sequence - Reverse sequence can occur with TFCC or DRUJ injury starting with luno triquetral ligament

Carpal instability adaptive - Dorsal angulation radius so distal row must flex, overloads SLL resulting in disruption → SLAC wrist

Q14. What are SLAC and SNAC wrists?

Scapholunate Advanced Collapse (SLAC), Scaphoid Nonunion Advanced collapse (SNAC)

Watson stages are essentially same for both:
1) **Radial styloid OA** - radial styloidectomy with or without PIN AIN neurectomy
2) **Radioscaphoid OA** - proximal row carpectomy
3) **Lunato-capitate OA** - 4 corner / wrist fusion
4) **Pan carpal OA** - may involve lunate fossa 4 corner / wrist fusion

Q15. How would you treat Keinbocks disease?

Lichtman stage and ulnar variance define treatment.

Stage 1 - MRI / bone scan changes - 3 months casting
Stage 2 - Lunate sclerosis, fracture lines - Plus **radial** shortening / bone graft
Stage 3 - Lunate collapse
  3A Normal alignment & height - Vascularized bone grafting
  3B Fixed rotation scaphoid (ring sign) - STT SC fusion or PRC
Stage 4 - Severe collapse OA at midcarpal or radiocarpal joints - PRC / fusion

Q16. Base of thumb arthritis stages and treatments?

Eaton Classification:
Stage 1 joint wide – inj / scope / ext osteotomy / recon ligament FCR 'Eaton'
Stage 2 <2mm osteophytes and sclerosis – trapeziectomy or fusion
Stage 3 >2mm osteophytes, narrow – fuse / replace or trapeziectomy
Stage 4 pan trapaezio arthrosis - fuse in 30 deg abduction 30 ext 15 pronation

Q17. Chronic regional pain syndrome / reflex sympathetic dystrophy?

Type 1 no nerve injury **Type 2** nerve injury

Definition sustained sympathetic activity with pain out of proportion to physical exam

Lankford stages:
1. **Acute 0-3months** pain swelling warmth redness, dec ROM, sweating, normal xr positive bone scan (phase III hot)
2. **Subacute 3-12mth** osteopenia, increasing pain, cyanosis, skin atrophy
3. **Chronic >12mths** pain decrease, skin glossy, osteopenia, joint contractures, less sweating

Diagnosis – if sympathetic block removes pain, but clinical diag.

Treatments – physio, alpha-blockers, antidepressants, antiepileptics, Ca channel blockers, GABA agonists, chemical or surgical sympathectomy, nerve stimulators.

Q18. Zones of flexor tendon injury?

Verdan zones

I	- Distal to FDS
II	- FDS to palmar crease
III	- Occurs between the distal palmar crease + stops at carpal tunnel
IV	- Carpal tunnel
V	- Carpal tunnel to musculotendinous junction

Q19. Compartment syndrome of the hand, how would you deal with it?

10 compartments in the hand:

4 dorsal interosseous, 3 volar interosseous, thenar hypothenar and carpal tunnel

Technique:
1. Incise 2nd + 4th MC + adductor thumb dorsally
2. Thenar and hypothenar via incision over 1st and 5th MC volar surface
3. Release carpal tunnel – then close skin by 10days if cannot then skin graft

Q20. Do you have a rehab protocol for flexor tendon injury?

Strickland early active motion protocol 1990s:
0-4wks tenodesis splint with passive ROM exercises between tenodesis exercises
4wk remove dorsal block during exercise but no wrist and finger extension at same time
5wk **active** excursion finger exercise
6wk blocking / isolation exercises
7wk passive extension
8wk resistance exercises

Q21. What is Quadriga syndrome?

Loss of flexion of an adjacent normal finger following limitation of proximal excursion of the FDP tendon of the injured digit. The patient typically complains of weakness in an inability to grasp with the injured and non-injured digits.

Q22. Kanavel signs flexor tenosynovitis?

1) Fusiform swelling of the involved digit (sausage digit)
2) Semi flexed position of the finger
3) Severe tenderness with palpation along the course of the tendon sheath
4) Excruciating pain with passive extension of the finger

Q23. *Dupuytren cords and contractures?*

1) **Central** — MCP contracture
2) **Spiral** — PIPJ contracture
3) **Lateral** — DIPJ contracture
4) **Natatory superficial TML** superficial palmar fascia contracture
5) **Abduct digiti mini**
6) **Commissural** (1st web)

Q24. *Describe the course of the median nerve?*

Proximal to distal:
- Medial to the brachial artery, anterior surface of **brachialis**.
- Between two heads of the **pronator teres**
- Between **FDS & FDP**
- Supplies the **pronator teres, FCR, PL, FDS** and <u>lumbricals</u> (radial)
- AIN → between **FPL** and the **FDP**. It supplies the radial half of the **FDP, FPL**, and the **pronator quadratus.**

Median Nerve in the forearm is found between **FDS** and **FCR**. Gives off:
1) **Palmer cutaneous branch** proximal to TCL
2) **Recurrent motor branch** at TCL thenar muscles and radial lumbricals.
3) **Common digital nerve** for the **thumb & digital nerve**

Q25. *Describe where the nerve can be compressed?*

1) supracondylar process
2) ligament of struthers
3) bicipital aponeurosis
4) ulnar and humeral heads of pronator teres
5) fds – confused with carpal tunnel –involves palmar cutaneous branch

Examination: Worse with resisted pronation with elbow extended or supination and resisted flexion (bicip apon) or resisted fds. 80% success decompress all 5.

Q26. *Describe the course of the radial nerve?*

Radial nerve:
- Between **brachialis - brachioradialis**
- Gives off the PIN, superficial radial sensory b/w **brachioradialis** and **ECRL**
- PIN moves under the **ECRB** and between the two heads of the **supinator**.

Q27. *Describe where the radial nerve can be compressed?*

1) Radio capitellar joint
2) ECRB- **middle finger extension diagnosis for compression of radial nerve**
3) Froshe (supinator proximal) – **resisted supination**
5) Henry (radial artery vessel leash)
6) Supinator distal – **resisted supination**

Q28. *Describe where the ulnar nerve can be compressed?*

1) Arcade of Struthers
2) Intermuscular septum
3) Exostosis medial epi
4) Osbourne's fascia
5) Accessory muscle anconeus
6) FCU distally

Q29. *Describe the boarders of the cubital tunnel?*

- Olecranon, medial epicondyle, Osborne ligament, MCL

Q30. What are the anatomical boundaries of Guyon's?

- **Roof** carpal ligament (VCL) and palmaris brevis
- **Floor** TCL, opponens digiti minimi
- **Ulnar wall** FCU, pisiform, and AbDM
- **Radial wall** Extrinsic flexor tendons, hook of the hamate

Q31. Median nerve palsy, what can you use to restore function?

- **Palmaris / proprius / FDS (long/ring)** to abd.p.b (FPL can then oppose the thumb)
- **Brachioradialis** to FPL
- **ECRL** to index **FDP**

Q32. Ulnar nerve palsy what can you use to restore function?

- **Split FDS** to re-create the **lumbrical function** – reattach to the base of each proximal phalanx or conjoined lateral bands.
- To **restore thumb adduction** – use ECRB or ring finger FDS.
- Suture **FDP** tendons to the other FDP tendons for finger flexion

Q33. Radial nerve palsy what can you use to restore function?

- **ECRL ECRB** and **brachioradialis** can be used or **FCR FCU** – if low palsy
- Loss of wrist extension → trans Teres to ECRB (if it's gone),
- **Finger extension FCU** to **EDC.**
- **Thumb extension** or abduction →trans **palmaris longus.**

Q34. Where are the pulleys?

- **5 Annular pulleys** A1, A3, and A5 are at the level of the MP, PIP, and DIP joints = volar plate.

- **A2 and A4** mid P1 and mid P2.
- Between each annular pulley after A2 is a C pulley eg: A2 - C1, A3 - C2.

Q35. Dorsal compartments of the wrist?

1. **APL (two slips) & EPB (always ulnar)** - DeQuervain
2. **ECRL & ECRB** - Intersection syndrome & tenosynovitis
3. **EPL** - Tenosynovitis & rupture
4. **EDC& EIP(ulnar) & PIN (sensory)** - Stenosing synovitis
5. **EDM** - Absent in 50%
6. **ECU** - Subluxation of ECU associated with TFCC

Q36. What is a lumbrical plus hand?

Lumbrical plus (intrinsic tightness) finger describes paradoxical extension of the interphalangeal joints when attempting to flex the involved digit.

Q37. Do we have any surgical options for distal radio ulnar joint OA?

- **Darrach** - Distal ulnar resection
- **Bowers hemi resection-interposition arthroplasty** Excision of articular surface of ulnar head DRUJ Preserve ulnar attachments to TFCC, minimizing postoperative instability
- **Sauve-Kapandji** - Radioulnar joint fusion
- **Ulnar arthroplasty**

Q38. What is Rheumatoid arthritis?

- Autoimmune systemic disease T cell mediated
- **IgM** (abnormal **Rh** antibody) attacks **native IgG** antibody
- Immune complex deposition allows monocyte mediated destruction of normal tissues

Q39. What are the orthopaedic manifestations?

- Progressive joint destruction instability and arthritis
- **Tenosynovitis** and subsequent rupture EDM, EDC, EPL **(Vaughan-Jackson)**
- **Caput ulnae syndrome** is chronic DRUJ synovitis ECU sublux → wrist instability
- **Synovitis causing PIN compression (elbow)** – test with tenodesis effect = MCPJ should extend with wrist flexion if tendons are intact

Q40. How can you treat multiple tendon ruptures?

- Address the **DRUJ** & <u>**tenosynovectomy**</u>
- **1 rupture** - repair - suture to adjacent tendon - tendon graft
- **2 ruptures** add in EIP transfer
- **3 or 4 ruptures** add in FDS transfer or FCR

Q41. ATLS approach to major burns after ABCDE?

- Consider fasciotomies of all compartments / escharotomies and serial debridement
- **Burn = 48 deg injury** ATLS 2-4ml x wt x % burn in 24hrs fluids
- Percentage area estimates using 1% 9% 18% areas

Q42. What should you consider / principles of tendon transfer – SSSSSSSS (8 S's)

- Supple (joint mobility)
- Strength (MRC grade 5)
- Sacrifice (gain more than loss)
- Synergy (appropriate)

- Stability
- Single (one motor per joint)
- Sensibility (not to a neuropathic area)
- Straight line of pull

Q43. *Surgical approach to the anterior forearm?*

- Incision from biceps to radial styloid. Nervous plane is between brachioradialis and FCR distally and pronator teres proximally
- **Superficial** layer is 4 muscles pronator teres, FCR, Palmaris longus, FCU
- **Middle layer** is FDS
- **Deep** is FDP pronator quadratus and FPL

Q44. *Surgical approach to the posterior forearm?*

- Incision is from lateral epicondyle to listers tubercle
- Separate **EPL** and **ECRB** to expose radius distally
- Proximally need to identify the PIN as it comes out of the supinator and dissect this out of the muscle to get at this part of the radius **b/w two most lateral muscles in the wad = ECRL and EDC (Kaplan approach to elbow – PIN at risk here)**
- Can strip supinator off the bone here between ECRB and supinator – do this with the arm supinated to move the nerve away. In the mid third you encounter **AbPL** and **EPB** attached to radius – you can strip these prox or distally how you want or slide plate under them.
- PIN is in the midline on the interosseous membrane. It is joined by the **PI Artery**

Q45. *Volar approach to scaphoid and lunate?*

- Incision on ulnar side of thenar crease (curved) then a hump at the wrist crease then straight to palmaris longus

- Watch out for **palmar cutaneous branch of medial nerve** ulnar to FCR above palmaris longus and median nerve. Open TCL with palmaris longus to the medial ulnar side
- Take flexor tendon mass to the ulnar side, median nerve radial side
- Expose scaphoid and lunate

Q46. Surgical technique to wash out a flexor sheath infection?

- Transverse incision at A1 pulley (MTPJ – palmer crease) – open it if pus found – open distal sheath with lateral incision or Z incision and wash out

Chapter 9: Shoulder & Elbow

Q1. *Blood supply to the shoulder from the axillary artery?*

Pectoralis minor divides the **axillary artery** into 3 parts:
- 1st part (pre) supreme thoracic artery
- 2nd part (under) thoraco-acromial artery and lateral thoracic
- 3rd part (after) subscapular, ant and post humeral circumflex arteries

Q2. *Blood supply to the elbow?*

Profunda brachi artery splits into radial collateral – ant and post and anterior branch of profunda brachi (anastomosis at front of elbow with radial artery, brachial artery branches into ulnar collateral superior and inferior which branches into anterior and posterior branches (interosseous branches).

Q3. *Describe the delto-pectoral approach?*

Will need to displace conjoint tendon medially to access subscap – keep arm adducted and ext rotate to protect plexus. Initial incision is over coracoid and down delto-pec groove to humerus. Subscap can be taken off in ext rotation or internal rotation with a flake of bone. To extend and gain control of bleeding axillary vessels or brachial plexus incision moves to mid clavicle and middle 1/3. To extend distally run the incision down the lateral side of biceps – retract that medially – brachialis is right under this to be split straight down onto the humerus. **Anterior circumflex humeral artery** crosses just under deltoid at top part of where pec major inserts.

Q4. *Describe the posterior approach to the shoulder?*

Spine of scapula incision, between teres minor (axillary) and infraspinatus (suprascapular nerve). Frist detach deltoid off the scapula spine the incision between the above muscles.

Q5. Describe the anterior-lateral approach to the elbow (anterior really)?

Is a continuation of the deltopectoral approach distally (can extend distally and proximally). Distally just between brachioradialis and brachialis can identify the **radial nerve** and **lateral antebrachial cutaneous nerve** at the elbow between these two muscles. Can extend distally between pronator teres and brachioradialis into the Henry approach to forearm.

Can modify this as a direct anterior approach S incision curved over medial side of biceps. Identify **lat cutaneous nerve** of forearm between brachialis and brachioradialis then biceps aponeurosis. **Radial artery** is right under the aponeurosis lateral to the **median** nerve with is lateral to the **brachial artery**. Pronator teres and biceps can be moved medially and brachioradialis laterally. Supinate to take off supinator and then onto joint capsule.

Q6. Describe the posterior approach to the elbow?

Posterior approach – triceps has two layers – lateral head from the lateral tip of the spiral groove and the long head from infra glenoid tubercle (outer layer). The inner layer is the medial head between the two is the **prof brachi artery** and **radial nerve**. Ulnar nerve is vulnerable deep to the medial head, incision can be extended distally over elbow. Cannot extend proximally past spiral groove.

Q7. Describe the lateral approach to the elbow to fix a lateral condyle fracture?

Lateral approach – incision along lateral supracondylar ridge between brachioradialis and triceps lateral head. Will encounter the common extensor origin distally ECU and anconeus (PIN and radial nerve supply) which can be elevated or extended through distally to gain access to radial head and joint. **Radial nerve** is there at intermuscular septum.

Q8. Describe the medial approach to the elbow to fix a medial condyle fracture?

Medial approach humerus – proximally brachialis and triceps long head and distally between brachialis and pronator teres which becomes common flexor origin distally. Before deep fascia is encountered branches of **medial cutaneous nerve** of the forearm are seen crossing distal incision (neuroma risk). Then medial epicondyle osteotomy to get into the joint if required → will allow access to the coronoid where brachialis inserts.

Q9. Slap tests?

Yergason test Resisted supination of the forearm with the elbow slightly flexed

Speed test Resisted forward elevation of the arm with the elbow extension and supination

O' Brien sign Pain with resisted downward force on the arm in an adducted (10 degrees) and 90-degree forward-flexed, maximally internally rotated shoulder. This pain may be relieved if the arm is brought into external rotation and supination.

Q10. Describe outcomes for shoulder replacements?

Radnay (JSES) meta-analysis >1900 = total shoulder gives better revision rates 6.5% comp to 10% for hemi/resurface at 5years, better ROM, better pain relief.

Q11. *What are the stages of adhesive capsulitis in the shoulder?*

Hannafin (CORR) stages:
- **Stage 1** (3months) *painful* stage no loss of motion
- **Stage 2** (3-9mth) *freezing* stage pain, loss of passive motion
- **Stage 3** (9 -15mths) *frozen* little pain mainly loss of motion
- **Stage 4** (>15mths) *thawing* phase little pain but improvement in motion.

Q12. *How can you classify a cuff tear?*

1) **Location** i.e. bursal, joint side or intra-substance
2) **Size (Codman)**: small <1cm, medium 1-3cm, large 3-5cm, massive >5cm
3) **Configuration: C shaped** (central tendon mass gives way), **U** shaped (more central retractions**), L shaped** (tear held with single limb), **reverse L** shaped or **complete**. Repair side to side (margin convergence) and end to bone.

Q13. *How can we reduce a shoulder dislocation / evidence?*

- **Stimson method** 4.5kg suspended from the arm (shoulder reduction)
- **Rockwood method** hypocratic method with sling around upper body
- **Hovileus (JBJS)** found the very re high dislocation rates for young patients
- **Itoy (JSES)** controversial study regarding bracing and external rotation

Q14. *Can you classify SLAP tears of the shoulder?*

Snyder:
- **Type I:** degeneration of superior glenoid labrum.

- **Type II**: detachment of superior glenoid labrum with biceps tendon attached
- **Type III**: bucket-handle type tear of labrum with biceps ok
- **Type IV**: Lengthwise tear of biceps tendon in which one part remains attached to the labrum and the other part attached to the tubercle.

Q15. *What is thoracic outlet syndrome, clinical tests?*

Definition: neurovascular compressive neuropathy
Provocation tests, WAR! Wright & Addison tests for vascular, Roos test for neuro:
- **Wright** – abduction and external rotation - neck rotated away (Loss of pulse and causes symptoms = positive)
- **Addison (adduct the head towards the arm 'Addison' – with 'air' taking a deep breath)** – extend arm neck extended and towards the effected side this time with patient taking a deep breath in.
- **Roos (neuro)** – open close hand in the surrender position 1 min.

Q16. *What is quadrilateral space syndrome?*

Compression between teres minor (axillary nerve), major (superior and inf subscapular nerves), long head triceps and humerus, **post circumflex humeral artery** and **axillary nerve** compressed.

Q17. *What types of elbow instability to you know?*

Valgus instability: Moving valgus stress test 100% sensitive 76% specific for UCL medial injury – looking for pain or apprehension or instability = positive test for this in clinic. >3mm opening on stress radiographs for diagnosis.

Posterior lateral rotatory instability: (usually coronoid tip fracture, radial head fracture and LCL injury – dislocation = **terrible triad injury**) **traumatic**, combination of supination, axial load and valgus causes the initial injury and is also the test for the condition (starting in extension). Results in post subluxation or radial head.

Varus posteromedial rotatory instability—Results from a fracture of the **anteromedial coronoid** process and **LUCL** injury. Treatment requires **ORIF** of the coronoid and LUCL reconstruction.

Q18. Anatomical structures stabilizing the elbow?

CAL – primary: coronoid, ant band of MCL and LCL
CAR – secondary: capsule, anconeus, radial head

Chapter 10: Paediatric Genetics & Dysplasia

Q1. How do the limbs form in an embryo?

- 4 weeks limb buds made of mesoderm and ectoderm –limb and joint formation
- 8 weeks nutrient artery appears, primary intra memb ossification occurs
- Continues circumferentially around each bone
- In the epiphyseal region enchondral ossification occurs
- At 9 weeks limbs begin to rotate towards their normal anatomical position
- 12 weeks all ossification centres in long bones formed
- At end of foetal development secondary ossification centres form initially in the distal femur and proximal femur at 3 months of age.

Q2. What kinds of congenital limb abnormalities do you know?

Swanson classified limb congenital abnormalities into 7 groups *(Mnemonic F DOSH CD)*

F = failure of formation
D = duplication
O = overgrowth
S = segmentation
H = hypertrophy
C = constriction rings
D = dysplasia syndromes

Q3. Do you know any specific mutations for genetic conditions?

Musculoskeletal Disorder	Genetic Mutation
Achondroplasia	FGF receptor 3
Osteogenesis imperfecta	Type I collagen

Pseudo achondroplasia	Cartilage oligomeric matrix protein (COMP)
Marfan syndrome	Fibrillin
Spondyloepiphyseal dysplasia	Type II collagen
Multi epiphyseal dysplasia	COMP
Diastrophic dysplasia	Sulphate transporter
Duchenne dystrophy	Dystrophin
X-linked hypoPO4 rickets	PEX endopeptidase
Osteopetrosis	Carbonic anhydrase
Fibrous dysplasia	G receptor protein
Multiple hereditary exostosis	EXT1 EXT2 EXT3 genes

Q4. Are there any clinical features common to all skeletal dysplasia's?

1) Relative hypertelorism
2) Short stature
3) Short limbs (rhizomelic)
4) Dysmorphic face
5) Spine scoliosis +/- stenosis +/- instability c spine
6) Stiff joints
7) Angular deformity of lower limbs - other than spine ones which don't!

Q5. What is achondroplasia?

- 1 in 30,000 to 50,000
- Autosomal dominant but 80% area new spontaneous mutations of FGF3
- Standard features of dysplasia's with hypermobility
- **Cartilaginous proliferative zone of the physis** is affected
- Foramen magnum stenosis is common
- Hydrocephalus, stenosis is common lumbar and foramen magnum, kyphosis and craniocervical instability champagne glass pelvis
- **Hypochondroplasia & Pseudo achondroplasia** less common less severe

Q6. *What is Hereditary Multiple Exostoses?*

- Skeletal dysplasia effects 1 in 18,000
- Autosomal dominant condition exostosin (EXT) genes
- Effects hips knees and ankles with valgus asymmetric shortening of limbs

Q7. *What is a mucopolysaccharidoses?*

- Deficiency of specific lysosomal enzymes result in accumulation of partially degraded glycosaminoglycans
- Effects 1 in 25,000 live births
- Common clinical features of skeletal dysplasia + organomegaly, cardiac problems.
- All are autosomal recessive except Hunters (X linked)
- Diagnosis by skin fibroblast biopsy genetic profiling

MPS I &V	**Hurler** syndrome
MPS II	**Hunter** disease
MPS III	**Sanfilippo** syndrome
MPS IV	**Morquio** syndrome joint laxity

Q8. *Tell me about multiple epiphyseal dysplasia (Trevor's disease)?*

- Delayed epiphyseal ossification, multi epiphyseal osteochondroma
- Mild short stature, limb deformities (may not see), and early-onset osteoarthritis
- Autosomal dominant with standard dysplasia clinical features
- Contractures of knees and elbows
- XR pelvis can look like **bilateral Perthes** *(classic exam question)*

Q9. *Tell me about the orthopaedic issues with Downs Syndrome?*

- Effects 1 in 1000 (trisomy 21)
- Celiac disease, Hirschsprung disease, gastroesophageal reflux, epilepsy, blood disorders (AML), abnormal thyroid function, and cardiac anomalies (endocardial cushion defects)
- Orthopaedic problems are scoliosis, SUFE, patellar instability, flat foot, metatarsus primus varus, and most importantly, atlantoaxial instability
- ADI 10 mm with no neurologic symptoms are observed yearly, stabilization for symptomatic ADI between 5 and 10 mm or >10mm.

Q10. *Tell me about* Osteogenesis Imperfecta?

- Type I collagen defect chromosome 17, AR and AD types
- Fractures heal at a normal rate
- Scoliosis and protrusio
- Long bones thin and bowed multiple old fractures

Sillence classification:

I most common, mild to moderate bone fragility, little or no deformity **Blue sclera (AD)**

II lethal in infancy fragile bones, severe deformity, perinatal **Blue sclera (AR)**

III moderate to severe deformity, progressive, fractures **(AR)**

IV moderately severe, long bone/spine deformity **(AD)**

Q11. *What is Perthes of the hip?*

- AVN of the immature hip
- Incidence 1 in 9000, M:F 4:1

- Usually thin, active, boy, social class 4 or more aged 4 or more
- Typically, short stature and delayed bone age by 2 years, bilateral in 15%

Causes:
1) Repeated ischaemic episodes and bone remodelling
2) Hydrostatic pressure and venous occlusion
3) Fibrinolytic disorders (Protein S & C, factor V, anticardiolipin antibody)
4) Passive smoking (social class)

Stages (Waldenstrom's)
1) **osteonecrotic infarction** (sclerosis) - 1ˢᵗ sign
2) **fragmentation** (pillar stages) 1 year - *so may be up to a year before can classify which is a major problem when you have lack of time i.e. age >8yrs*
3) **resorption** via **creeping substitution + re ossification** 3-5yrs
4) **remodelling**

Herring classification = strongest predictor of outcome
- C group 1/8th will have good outcome
- B/C = 50% height group 1/4ᵗʰ will have a good result#
- B group 2/3ʳᵈ will have good result
- A group (normal lateral pillar) nearly all will have a good result

Q12. What influences surgical decision making in Perthes?

- Based on (1) age (2) grade and (3) stage
- Bracing – ok for pain relief but does not alter natural progression
- **Herring (JBJS)** study on >400 patients
- **6 years** or less no evidence that anything you do makes a difference#
- **>6years** consider containment for all but A's with salters or varus osteotomy if head at risk signs

Q13. What did the paper actually say about surgical management?

- <8yrs and B or more surgery made no difference but actually it <u>DID</u> in their paper as non-op group outcome was 25% good vs >60% good in op group so probably under powered!...
- The alternative (deciding not to contain the head) is you wait to see if the patient is an A or a C in the >8yrs group but if you do you wait you miss the boat.

Q14. What are the 'head at risk' signs?

Catterall's head at risk signs:
L = Lytic area in lateral epiphysis = **gage** sign V shape = hinge abduction
C = Calcification lateral to femoral head epiphysis = ossification of extruded head
S = ***Subluxation (most important)*** – caused by thick cartilage medially on the femoral head and acetabulum causing mushrooming of the head
M = Metaphyseal reaction – indicates non-ossified areas of cartilage in the growth plate – areas of lucency under growth plate = cysts
G = Growth plate in horizontal position indicating the hip is in external rotation

Q15. How can we predict outcome in a mature femoral head?

Stullberg classification (JBJS) – predict OA changes **at maturity**

Type 1	Normal
Type 2	Spherical head but coxa magna and short neck coxa brevis = no early OA
Type 3	Mushroom = **mild** early OA
Type 4	Flat – but! Joint same shape as head – congruent joint = **moderate chance of** OA

Type 5   Both side of the joint incongruent with flat head =
           OA risk severe

This demonstrates that **sphericity** *and* **congruence** are both important

Q16. *Surgical containment options?*

- **Femoral varus osteotomy** (good 8-10 years)
- **Salter pelvic osteotomy** (good >6yrs)
- **Shelf / Chiari** – large incongruent joint = non-re-directional (older patient)

Q17. *What are the risk factors for hip dysplasia?*

- **Female**
- **First born**
- **Fam Hx**
- **Feet first (breech)**
- **Foot deformity**

Q18. *When is a Pavlik harness appropriate?*

Effective up to 6months. Can be used for dislocated hips but should stop if not reduced in 3weeks. Hip flexion 100 abduction 50 deg = **safe zone** of **Ramsey**. Worn 23 hours a day for at least 6 weeks after a reduction has been achieved and then an additional 6 weeks part-time (nights and naps).

Q19. *What are the potential obstructions to reduction?*

- Iliopsoas tendon
- Pulvinar
- Contracted inferomedial hip capsule
- Transverse acetabular ligament

- Inverted labrum
- Hypertrophic ligamentum teres

Q20. What are your options when a harness is inappropriate (6months +)?

- **Closed reduction**: 6 to 18 months. arthrogram to assess reduction, and hip spica
- **Open reduction**: 6 to 18 months and fail closed reduction, have an obstructive limbus, or have an unstable safe zone. Open reduction is also the **initial treatment for children 18 months** and older. It is usually done through an anterior approach, especially for patients older than 12 months (less risk to the **medial femoral circumflex artery**) and includes capsulorrhaphy, adductor tenotomy, femoral shortening to take tension off the reduction, and an acetabular procedure if severe dysplasia is present.
- Diagnosis after age 8 years (younger in patients with bilateral DDH) may contraindicate reduction because the acetabulum has little chance to remodel, although reduction may be indicated in conjunction with salvage procedures.

Q21. What causes a SUFE?

Slipped capital femoral epiphysis: weakness of the perichondral ring and slippage through the hypertrophic zone of the growth plate. The femoral head remains in the acetabulum, and the neck is displaced anteriorly and externally rotates. On physical examination, all patients have obligated external rotation with flexion of the hip. Incidence is 3-7 per 100,000, 3:1 male, 30% bilateral.

Q22. Xray signs of SUFE?

1) Loss of Klein's line (Trethowan sign)
2) Metaphyseal blanch of steel (crescent density in metaphysis) = overlap due to slip
3) Joint space increase inferiorly

4) Wide/wooly/irregular density change in physis
5) Decreased epiphyseal height (due to slip)
6) Remodeling changes inferiorly medially due to callus formation.

Q23. *What influences surgical management?*

Loder's stability classification 0% osteonecrosis in stable slips - can wt bear with or without crutches stable = **no surgery**, 47% of the patients with unstable slips developed AVN = **surgery**.

Southwick slip angle – angle on lateral xray (head shaft angle minus normal sides angle)
- Type I: 30deg   - fix in situ
- Type II: 30-60deg   - fix in situ
- Type III: >60deg   - may need cuneiform osteotomy to reduce (specialist centre)

Technique:
- **Jusanti (JBJS)** 6.4mm screws 3 threads required to maintain fixation
- **Peterson (JPO)** Reduction performed <24hrs = 7% AVN, >24hrs = 20% AVN, so if not done in 24hrs → skin traction for up to 3wk then fix (lowers rate of AVN)

Chapter 11: Neuromuscular Paediatrics

Q1. *What is Scheuermanns Disease?*

- Increased **thoracic kyphosis with 5 degrees** or more of anterior wedging at **three** sequential levels. Greater than 45 deg kyphosis on extension radiograph
- Incidence is 1-8% **AD**, usually 8-12yrs, male, can be **type 1** (thoracic) or **type 2** (lumbar) - brace patients until mature
- Curves >**75 degrees = Posterior fusion to include the 1st lordotic disc to prevent junctional kyphosis** to correct to at least 50 deg (max extent of normal

Q2. *Neurofibromatosis?*

- Incidence 1 in 5000, **AD** but 50% new mutations Chromosome 17
- **NF1 (peripheral type -** *Von Reckinghausans disease*)
- **NF2 (central type)** with bilateral vestibular schwannoma's

7 Diagnostic criteria – patient must have at least 2:
1) 1st deg relative (as its **AD**)
2) 2 iris hamartomas (lish nodules)
3) 3 different lesions (either 2 neurofibroma or 1 plexiform neurofibroma)
4) Freckles in axillary or inguinal region
5) Optic glioma
6) 6 or more café – au – lait spots
7) Distinctive osseous lesion associated with NF eg sphenoid dysplasia or thinning of long bone cortex with or without pseudarthrosis

Q3. *Tell me about Charcot-Marie-Tooth Disease?*

Is part of a larger group of hereditary **motor sensory** neuropathies (HMSN). There are X linked, AR and AD forms.

HMSN I is **AD** Chromosome 17 myelin protein, motor/sensory **demyelinating** neuropathy - **hypertrophic** and has an onset during the **second** decade of life

HMSN II is **neuronal** causing direct axonal death by **Wallerian degeneration**, less disabling. Variable inheritance, onset **third** decade more foot involvement.

Clinical features: intrinsic wasting in the hands. The most severely affected muscles are the tibialis anterior, peroneus longus, and peroneus brevis. Motor defects > sensory defects. Pes cavus, hammer toes with frequent corns/calluses, peroneal weakness, and "stork legs." Low nerve conduction velocities with prolonged distal latencies are noted in peroneal, ulnar, and median nerves.

Diagnosis is made most reliably by **DNA testing** for chromosome 17

Q4. *Paediatric spine deformity, classification?*

1) Congenital (bars /hemivertebra – failure of **segmentation/formation/ mixed**)
2) Idiopathic (infantile, child, adolescent)
3) Neuromuscular scoliosis

Infantile idiopathic scoliosis (< 3 yrs) apical rib–vertebral angle difference (RVAD) of Mehta. Curves less than 25 degrees with an RVAD less than 20 degrees tend to resolve spontaneously, observation – if more consider operation.

Juvenile idiopathic scoliosis (3 - 10 yrs), high risk of curve progression operate at adolescent growth spurt if possible or **at 50deg.**

Adolescent idiopathic scoliosis (10 yrs) Bracing for Cobb angles <u>**up to 45 deg,**</u> is only effective in **skeletally immature** patients and **will not correct deformity** but may **prevent progression** in a **flexible curve (up to Reisser grade II).**
- **Posterior** fusion for **>45 deg Cobb**
- **Anterior+posterior** fusion for larger curves and stiff curves >75deg and to prevent crankshaft in girls <10 boys <12yrs + Risser grade 0.

Fusion rules (always must have progression +/- always consider to pelvis or not):
- **Neuromuscular/duchenns** from **30deg (as will progress at growth spurt)**
- **<3 infantile** consider from **35deg**
- **3-10 juvenile** consider from **50deg**
- **>10 adolescent** consider at growth spurt if **>45deg**
- **Congenital with hemi bar / hemi vert** that will progress at any point
- **T2-sacrum** for neuro
- Add in **anterior** to prevent crankshaft if boys <12 girls <10, Risser 0
- Fuse to a **neutral vertebra** or 1 level above and 2 below **end vertebra**

Q5. *What is the Risser grade along the iliac crest?*

Rissers 0-5: 0 = no visible epiphysis, then in 25% increments 1-4 with 5 being fused.

Curve progression - 4 groups
Risser's 2 or more + < 20 deg curve = <2%
Risser's 2 or more + >20 deg curve = 23%
Risser's 0 or 1 < 20 deg curve = 22%
Risser's 0 or 1 >20 deg curve = 68% progression (operate)

Definitions (scoliosis research society) and principles:
- **Avoid** fusing below L3 and certainly L4 (back pain)
- **Stable** vertebra is first bisected by the central sacral vertical line

- **Neutral** vertebra = the one which is rotationally neutral i.e. tips
- **End vertebra** = vertebra with distal end plate maximally angulated
- **Lowest instrumented vertebra** one or two levels proximal to the stable vertebra or distal end vertebra.

Q6. *What is the clinical triad for Klippel Feil?*

1) Low hair line
2) Fusion of 2 or more vertebrae c spine
3) Short neck – associated with facial asymmetry, neck webbing, Sprengel shoulder

* Avoid contact sports → decompress / fusion for cervical instability

Q7. *Cerebral palsy – principles of orthopaedic management?*

- Avoid surgery in the first 3 years of life unless hip at risk
- **Selective dorsal root rhizotomy**: reduce spasticity
- **Hip dislocation - Reimers** migration index
- **Hip at risk** - reduced abduction, partial uncovering of the femoral head (Reimers >30% uncovered)
- Consider adductor tenotomy in children with abduction <20 degrees +/- psoas release/recession
- Femoral or pelvic osteotomies for dysplasia
- For patients over 4 yrs soft tissue procedures are not going to work alone
- **Spastic dislocation**: Consider open reduction, femoral shortening, varus derotation osteotomy, Dega's, triple, or Chiari's osteotomy

Q8. *What types of CP exist?*

1) **Spastic** 75%

2) **Athetoid/Dyskinetic** -slow, writhing, involuntary movement due to involvement of ***basal ganglia***- dysarthria; abnormal, distal, jerky
3) **Ataxic** balance and co-ordination, unsteadiness, a wide-based gait, and intentional tremor
4) **Hemi ballistic** violent, uncoordinated, involuntary movement
5) **Hypotonic**
6) **Mixed**

Q9. What is spasticity?

Velocity dependent increase in tone due to loss of inhibitory control of anterior horn cells.

Q10. What is 'GMFC' in relation to cerebral palsy?

GMFC (Gross motor function classification 1-5)
1 = walking
2 = walking with limits outdoors
3 = walking with aids indoor and out
4 = wheelchair self-powered
5 = electric wheelchair (no head control)

Chapter 12: Paediatric Trauma

Q1. Tell me what you know about brachial plexus palsy?

- 2 per 1000 births
- **Causes**: large baby, shoulder dystocia, forceps, breech position, and prolonged labour
- **Maintain passive ROM** and await return of motor function (up to 18 months)
- 90% resolve without intervention
- Lack of biceps function 6 months after injury / Horner's syndrome = poor prognosis
- Options include releasing contractures, latissimus and teres major transfer to the shoulder external rotators, tendon transfers for elbow flexion, proximal humerus rotational osteotomy, and microsurgical nerve grafting

Q2. Paedatric elbow fractures?

Lateral epicondyle # is <u>**less forgiving**</u> – may accept up to **2mm** displacement – high complications of AVN, malunion nonunion, ulnar nerve symptoms later on. **Medial epicondyle** can accept up to **5mm** as a painless fibrous union is not a problem.

Q3. Classifications of femoral fractures in children?

Delbert's femur classification I (AVN 40%) – II (30%) III – (20%) – IV (10%)

AAOS guidelines for femoral shaft fractures:
- **0-6mth** spica
- **6mth – 6 years** less than 3cm short = spica, if >3cm or open or polytrauma, mutlifragment = ORIF exfix, spica, or flexi nails
- **6-11years** with **length stable** (transverse or oblique pattern) flexi nail, **if length unstable fractures** (spiral, comminuted, very proximal very distal fracture) can use ORIF, exfix. 11yrs or approaching maturity if patients is <45kg and length stable fracture pattern use flexi nails, if the opposite then treat as adult
- **Mettazaeu formula** – multiply 0.4mm by canal size, goal is 80% canal fill. 2 nails of equal size are inserted retrograde 2cm above distal femoral physis. Removal at 1 year. Healing 3months.

Q4. Tibial spine fracture classification in children?

Myers-McKeever:
I minimal / no displacement anterior margin
II have an elevation of the anterior portion with an intact posterior hinge
III displaced

Chapter 13: Paediatric Lower Limb

Q1. How do you examine the rotational profile of the paediatric lower limbs?

- Foot progression angle during gait – nonspecific rotation
- Femoral version with the patient prone – usually corrects by age of 10
- Thigh foot angle = tibial torsion (most common cause consider osteotomy if >6 years)
- Foot lateral boarder and medial crease = metatarsus adductus
- Leg length testing

Q2. Clubfoot?

- **Clubfoot** (*congenital talipes equinovarus*)
- 1 in 1,000 live births with a 2:1 predominance in males, 50% bilateral
- **Causes**: neuromuscular disorders, diastrophic dwarfism, arthrogryposis, tibial hemimelia, and myelomeningocele

Definition: *congenital misalignments of talo-calcaneo-navicular axis of the foot*

Q3. Describe the Ponseti technique?

- Weekly plaster changes for 6 to 8 weeks
- Initially, the cavus is corrected by **supination** of the forefoot
- Followed by **abduction** of the supinated forefoot. This manoeuvre is done with the fulcrum over the lateral aspect of the talar head

- Once the foot is abducted to 60 degrees, then the **equinus** is corrected with dorsiflexion of the foot
- A percutaneous tenotomy of the tendo-achilles is necessary in rigid equinus
- **Ponseti (JPO)** 89% success with good results at 30yrs. 70% require the tenotomy
- After complete correction = Denis-Browne bar shoe full time for 3 months (70-degree external rotation of the feet)
- Then an abduction shoe is required only during night time whilst child is walking from 1 year of age

Q4. *What can be done for resistant clubfeet?*

- Post-medial release is considered at 6 to 9 months
- Anterior tibial tendon transfer to the dorsum of the midfoot can be done
- The affected foot has less growth potential and is smaller than the contralateral foot
- Medial opening or lateral column shortening is preferred from 3 to 10 years of age
- After age 10, a triple arthrodesis is the appropriate procedure

Q5. *Classification of metatarsus adductus?*

Beck's heel bisector line on wt bearing AP xray – passes **through:**
- **Normal 2nd 3rd toe web space**
- **Mild** deformity 3rd – observe
- **Moderate** 3-4th – casting 3months → abd H lengthen and capsulotomy
- **Severe** 4th-5th – as above +/- bone correction (medial cuneiform opening wedge)

Berg classification:
- **Simple** – adductus alone
- **Complex** – adductus with lateral shift of midfoot
- **Skew** adductus with hindfoot valgus

- **Complex skew (*serpentine foot*)** + lateral shift of midfoot- all 3! (Bony procedure). 90% will resolve by 4yrs. May be associated with hip dysplasia

Q6. Vertical talus?

Rigid rocker bottom flat foot (navicular dislocated dorsally) – (**initially cast 3 months**):
1) **Hindfoot equinovalgus** = contracted TA and peroneal tendons (**z lengthen**)
2) **Midfoot dorsiflexion / abduction** = dislocated navicular (**reduce**)
3) **Contracture of extrinsic tendons** EHL EDL tib ant (**z lengthen**)
4) **Contracture of joints** TN subtalar CC TT (**release**)

Causes: 20% of these patients have a family history, arthrogryposis, diastematomelia, neuromuscular, chromosome abnormality, congenital oblique talus is the same thing but the talus reduces with forced plantarflexion (hence need stress views to ensure we are not dealing with this benign condition which only requires observation.

Prognosis 60-80% will have a stiff but functional foot.

Q7. Tarsal coalitions?

Tarsal Coalition: is **autosomal dominant,** failure of mesenchyme segmentation, coalition can be fibrous/cartilaginous/osseous, 50% bilateral, 2% population, 25% symptomatic.

Q8. What other types of tarsal coalitions do you know?

Talo-navicular (3-5 yrs of age)

Calcaneo-navicular (8-12yrs – when ossification of the bar occurs). Is associated with elongated anterior process of the calcaneus **"anteater" sign**

Talo-calcaneal (usually middle facet at 12yrs). May demonstrate **talar beaking** on the lateral view (does not denote degenerative joint disease) or irregular middle facet on Harris's axial view or **C sign**

Q9. How do they present and xray findings?

Clinical presentation: Painful flat foot with rigid hindfoot. **Canale (oblique xray)** hindfoot demonstrate the calcaneonavicular bar, while the **Harris (posterior subtalar joint xray)** view shows the talocalcaneal bar. Diagnosis is with CT or MRI.

Treat with immobilization for up to 6 weeks - talocalcaneal bar involving less than 50% of **total subtalar joint surfaces are** treated with excision of the bar, while those who have greater than 50% involvement are treated with fusions.

Q10. Congenital knee dislocations?

- **Type 1** hyper extended - observation
- **Type 2** sublux - casting
- **Type 3** dislocation tibia anterior – quads plasty and soft tissue correction before 6mth

Q11. Congenital flexible flatfoot, what is it and how do you treat?

Calcaneovalgus (flexible flatfoot) — 1 in 1000, associated with posterior-medial tibial bowing. Newborn condition associated with intrauterine positioning, dorsiflexed hindfoot, with eversion and abduction of the hindfoot that is passively correctable to neutral.

Treatment consists of passive stretching /casting and observation. Also seen with myelomeningocele at the L5 level due to muscular imbalance.

Q12. What other congenital foot positioning can occur?

Equinovarus – common with **spastic hemiplegia**, duchenns, neuromuscular, cerebral palsy, residual club foot, tibial hemimelia, **operatively** – TA lengthening, split tib post to peroneus brevis, split tib ant to cuboid (rancho) and TA lengthening or bone procedures eg osteotomy.

Equinovalgus – spastic **diplegia and quadriplegia**, fibula hemimelia (space out laterally so foot twists out laterally), deformity is midfoot abduction, heel valgus, equinus, bilateral, ligamentous laxity, weak tib post and tib ant, spasticity of the peroneal tendons and gastro-soleous.

Q13. What are the common causes of leg length inequality (paediatrics)?

1) Hemihypertrophy
2) Dysplasia's
3) PFFD – proximal focal femoral deficiency
4) Metabolic /Endocrine
5) Spasticity
6) Polio
7) Infection
8) Tumours
9) Trauma

Q14. Treatment options?

Final predicted inequality of less than 2 cm doesn't require any treatment, 2 to 5 cm can be dealt with epiphysiodesis of the longer leg, 5 to 7 cm could be treated with limb lengthening, and more than 7 cm with contralateral epiphysiodesis and ipsilateral lengthening.

Distraction osteogenesis (limb lengthening) follows **Ilizarov principles**: low energy metaphyseal corticotomy, stability, good biology, settling period of 5 days, followed by gradual distraction 1mm a day in 4 turns of the distractor to create the **regenerate**.

Q15. What techniques can estimate final leg length?

- **Mosley** data (straight line method from a graph)
- **Anderson-Green data** for distal femur and proximal tibial growth – predicted (**based on bone age Greulich atlas**) – requires 3 scanograms and will tell you predicted LLD and remaining growth
- **White's rule of thumb** estimation technique – hip grows 3mm year / distal femur 9mm year / proximal tibia 6mm year / distal tibia 5mm year

Chapter 14: Pathology

Q1. **What is a Mirel score?**

Technique to estimate risk of pathological fracture where a metastatic deposit is found:

Score 7 = 4%, 8 = 15%, score of 9 >33% risk of fracture over 1 year

Score	Pain	Location	Xray	Diameter involved
1	Mild	Upper limb	Blastic	1/3
2	Mod	Lower limb	Mixed	2/3
3	Severe	Peri trochanter	Lytic	>2/3

Q2. **How can you classify severity of primary bone tumors?**

Enneking described his benign and malignant lesions:

Type 1 (latent) chondroma non oss fibroma, EG, osteoid osteoma, enchondroma

Type 2 (active) ABC, blastoma, UBC, chrondromyxoid fibroma

Type 3 (aggressive) Giant cell tumors and above, can be I (low grade), II (high grade), and III (mets) with A (intracompartmental) or B (extra compartmental)

General rules of tumor
1) **Benign** lesions → curettage and graft.
2) **Marginal resection** is for neuroleioma, glomus, tumours, periosteal chondroma, nodular fasciitis.

3) **Intermediate lesions** (parosteal osteosarcoma, chordoma, chondrosarcoma, adamantinoma, squamous cell) – **wide resection** for these.
4) **DXT it's a met** or if **soft tissue sarcoma** (liposarcoma, desmoid, fibrosarcoma/MFH, angiosarcoma).
5) **Wide resection** and **chemotherapy** for osteosarcoma, MFH/fibrosarcoma, de differentiate chondrosarcoma,
6) **Risk of pulmonary mets** 15-25% for anything intermediate grade or above

Q4. *Tell me about osteoid osteoma?*

Age group: 5-30yrs 2:1 male female.
Classical location: proximal femur-tibia-spine, can resolve spontaneously over 3 years.
Histology: *nidus* (immature woven bone surrounded by osteoblastic rimming) and reactive bone on the outer surface with a sclerotic border, it is the same as an osteoblastoma only smaller. A blastoma is bigger, has more giant cells and higher recurrence rate of >15%.

Q5. *Tell me about osteosarcoma?*

Intramedullary osteosarcoma – HISTOLOGY lacy osteoid and **pleomorphic cells** (pleomorphic = everybody looks different – chondroblastic, giant cells, osteoblastic, fibroblastic), **Genetics**: Mutations in **RB** gene >60%, and **p53** gene >30%. **Prognosis 5yrs** 80%.

Parosteal osteosarcoma – more common in females. **Prognosis 5yrs** 96%, **Radiographic** – heavily ossified (lower grade), **HISTOLOGY** – some cellular atypia, can look like normal osseous trabecular to a certain degree with interspersed spindle cells.

Periosteal osteosarcoma an intermediate grade tumor, radiographic usually no involvement of the intramedullary canal, classical finding is the **sunburst hair on end** radiographic feature. **HISTOLOGY** – mixed osteoid with some high-grade features.

Telangiectatic osteosarcoma – must differentiate this from an ABC (radiographically looks the same), very aggressive tumor. **Prognosis 5yrs** 70% (with mets 20%), **HISTOLOGY** – looks like a bag of blood with pleomorphic cells, minimal osteoid.

Q6. What is the difference between an enchondroma and an osteochondroma?

Enchondroma (in the bone) – low grade, typical patient is > 30yrs chondroblasts escape into the metaphysis and proliferate, **popcorn** calcification **ring** calcification on rays, minimal erosion but may expand **HISTOLOGY** – lots of extracellular matrix, blue/grey hyaline cartilage, enchondral ossification can create lamella bone no aggressive features. Difficult to differentiate a chondrosarcoma **so** 6-12monthly xrays.

Osteochondroma (on the bone) – the stalk is ossified bone histologically the cap is cartilage, suspect malignancy if >2cm cap.

MHE – Multi hereditary exostosis (up to 10% sarcoma-change) associated with **EXT1-2-3 tumor suppressor genes**.

Q7. Do you know any chondral tumor?

Chondroblastoma < 30yrs, usually open physis, <2% will become aggressive and met, well circumscribed metaphyseal lytic lesions, looks like a giant cell tumor on xrays may have a sclerotic rim, may nor may not have calcification or cortical expansion. **HISTOLOGY** – chondroblasts in chicken wire / cobblestone arrangement & chondroid matrix.

Chondrosarcoma can be **low / high grade** or **de-differentiated** >30yrs so tend to be less aggressive lesions overall. Higher grades look more like osteosarcoma. **HISTOLOGY** has a low grade chondroid component **and** high-grade spindle cell similar to osteosarcoma.

Q8. What is a fibrosarcoma?

Malignant fibrous histocytoma (MFH) / Fibrosarcoma most common soft tissue sarcoma between 50-80years in adults, can arise from a bone infarct – Paget's – irradiated area. **Prognosis 5years 50%.** Painless mass, can become a pathological fracture, can be calcified can be destructive (xray non-diagnostic), **HISTOLOGY – pleomorphic spindle** and histocytes in a storiform pattern, chronic inflammatory cells, malignant multi nucleated giant cells **Treatment – radiation, chemo and resection.**

Q9. What is a chordoma?

The most common primary malignant spinal tumor in adults, sacrum coccyx, **malignant tumor of notochord origin**. **Prognosis** 50% 5 years survival, patients usually >50yrs, 50% palpable on rectal exam, 50% recurrence rate. **HISTOLOGY** – foamy vacuolated phisolipherous cells staining positive immunohistochemical diagnosis. **Treatment** – wide surgical excision plus radiation if no clear margin – or radiation in isolation.

Q10. What is the difference between a unicameral and aneurysmal bone cyst?

Unicameral and aneurysmal bone cyst (ABC) < 20-year-old patients. **Unicameral cyst** - fluid filled failure of bone formation, **active** if next to physis or **latent** if away from it, well demarcated lesion – xray may show a *'fallen leaf sign'*. **HISTOLOGY** – cyst with fibrous lining, containing giant cells, hemosiderin pigmentated cells. **Treatments** – injection with prednisolone / marrow injection and aspirations (multi). May need to curette and graft or fix if really large, try to avoid surgery if active - may cause growth arrests.

ABC – most common in the **spine** and in association with other **tumors** (**30%** of the time – NOF, giant cell, fibrous dysplasia, expansive, **metaphyseal, lytic, eccentric with bone septa bubble appearance**, thin rim of new bone at the rim, CT and MRI show **multi fluid levels, HISTOLOGY** – cyst, blood filled spaces with no endothelial lining, spindle cells, benign giant cells, some woven new bone.

Q11. What is fibrous dysplasia?

Failure of normal mineralization→ **soap bubble appearance on radiographs** - lytic lesions with margin of sclerotic bone or ground glass appearance. **HISTOLOGY** –looks like **Chinese** letters or **alphabet** soup due to fibroblast proliferation around islands of woven bone with no osteoblastic rimming. There is osteoid and woven bone is fibrous stroma (hence fibrous dysplasia). **Treatment = bisphosphonates** to decrease pain and bone turnover in **polyostotic** fibrous dysplasia, fix impending fractures.

Q12. What might 'look' like bone on an xray/bone forming lesions?

- **Lamellar bone** is rarely produced by tumour and is usually native host bone
- **Woven bone <u>with</u>** osteoblastic rimming is reactive and indicative of fracture callus, periosteal reaction, or myositis ossificans.
- **Woven bone** with <u>**no**</u> osteoblastic rimming is **neoplastic** – but could still be benign
- **With malignant spindle cell stroma** = osteosarcoma

Differential- *if its looks like bone on an xray*:
- Fracture callus
- Myositis ossificans
- Melorheostosis
- Muchmeyers (fibrous dysplasia ossificans progressiva)
- Hypertrophic ossification

- Bone infarcts
- Mets to bone (can be osteosclerotic)
- Osteoid osteoma
- Osteoblastoma
- Fibrous dysplasia
- Parosteal osteosarcoma
- Osteosarcoma
- Any chondroid lesion can form immature bone
- Infection

If its looks like *calcium*:
- Tumoral calcinosis (not bone just calcification really)
- MFH and liposarcoma can show calcification but not bone

Q13. What kind of tumor is an Ewing's sarcoma?

Ewing's (primitive neuroectodermal tumor) – p53 mutation, 11 22 translocations always present, 21 – 22 translocations in 10%. **HISTOLOGY** small round blue cells, monotonous, **pseudorosetts** (*circles of cells with necrotic centre*). Lots of nuclear material no cytoplasm cells, diagnosis is immunohisto staining. **Differential histologically** – (small round blue cells) can be neuroblastoma, eosinophilic granuloma, myeloma, leukaemia, lymphoma, Ewing. **Prognosis**: 30% 5 years

Q14. What is a Schwannoma and other nerve tumors?

Neurilemoma (Schwannoma) – can affect motor / sensory nerves (in the sheath), >30-year-old NF 2 gene mutation, rare malignant transformation, **HISTOLOGY Antoni** A structure (bundles of spindle cells) **Antoni** B structure (areas of less cellularity) and **verocay** body alignment (2 rows) **Treatment** – excise.

Malignant nerve sheath tumor (Neurofibrosarcoma / Malignant schwannoma) >30-year-old, associated with NF 1 gene **HISTOLOGY** spindle cells wavy nuclei similar to a fibrosarcoma **Treatment** - wide resection and pre-op radiation.

Neurofibroma – 20-40-year-old, peripheral tumor of the extremities can be part of **neurofibromatosis** chromosome 17 mutation NF1 AD. Can be **dermal** (single nerve fusiform swelling of nerve – don't become malignant) Plexiform (bag of worms) multi nerve bundles – pathognomic of neurofibromatosis can become malignant. **HISTOLOGY** fibroblasts, schwan cells, fibrocytes, mast cells, lymphocytes **Treatment** – excise with or without nerve grafting.

Neuroblastoma 1 in 100,000 incidence, **HISTOLOGY** rosette pattern small round blue cells, most common solid tumor of childhood.

Chapter 15: Adult Spine

Q1. Topographical landmarks according to levels of the C spine to plan your approach?

Hard palate	= Arch of Atlas C1
Mandible	= C2-3
Hyoid cartilage	= C3
Thyroid cartilage	= C4-5
First cricoid ring	= C6
Carotid tubercle	= C6 (anterior tubercle of the transverse process of C6),
Vertebra prominens	= C7
Scapula spine	= T3
Scapula tip	= T7
Umbilicus	= L3-4 disk space
Iliac crest	= L4-5 interspace
PSIS	= S2

Q2. Give me the anterior approach to the C spine C3-T1 levels?

Transverse from midline to lateral boarder of sternocleidomastoid at topographic level. **Facial VII** nerve supply platysma then **accessory XI** nerve supply sternocleidomastoid. Split **deep fascia** then **platysma** top to bottom then between strap muscles medially (**sternohyoid sternothyroid - C1-3**) and **sternocleidomastoid** laterally, go medial to **carotid sheath through pre-tracheal fascia** then through **prevertebral fascia** between **longus coli** muscles on front of vertebral body.

Specific problems:
- **Superior thyroid artery C3-** can divide & watch out for **superior laryngeal nerve.**
- **Inferior thyroid artery C6** -protect
- **Recurrent laryngeal nerve C6** between oesophagus and trachea -protect

- **Cervical trunk** is in front of longus coli prevertebral fascia laterally -protect

Q3. What is the 'normal curvature of the spine?

Cervical: lordosis **20-40 deg** – all have bifid spinous process and anterior tubercle except C7.
Thoracic: kyphosis **20-50 deg** facets **angled steeply at 60 degrees.**
Lumbar: lordosis **40-80 deg** -mammillary processes project posteriorly from the superior, facets are **angled above 60 deg**.

Q4. What are Lhermitte's sign and Spurling's test?

Both signs of spinal pathology. **Lhermitte**: neck flexion causing lightning-like sensation radiating down back caused by cervical stenosis; disk herniation; multiple sclerosis with posterior column dysfunction. **Spurling**: lateral flexion to the side and axial load → radicular pain.

Q5. Are there any signs of non-organic pathology in relation to the spine?

Waddell signs for nonorganic pathology **3 or more = poor surgical outcome**:

(1) Pain **out of proportion** to stimulus (example, light touch)
(2) Pain in a **nonanatomic distribution**
(3) **Exaggerated pain** response
(4) **Skin roll** test: roll skin between index and thumb and note radicular symptoms
(5) **Head compression**: apply 5 lbs. of load – any symptoms will be non-organic
(6) **Twist test**: patient standing with feet planted, examiner rotates torso left and right - symptoms are all non-organic
(7) **Flip test**: Perform sitting and supine SLR and note any difference in pain

Q6. *How would you classify spinal cord injury?*

ASIA classification & spinal cord injury:
- **Sensory** / **motor** / **neuro** level is lowest *normal* segment on both sides
- **Tracts** are descending motor (**lateral** and **ventral cortico-spinal tracts**).
- **Dorsal columns** fasciculus gracilis (medial) and cuneatus (lateral) – deep touch proprioception and vibration.
- **Lateral spinal thalamic** (pain and temperature)
- **Anterior spinothalamic** (light touch).
- **Syndromes – central cord (medium prognosis)** most common, elderly
- **Anterior cord (worst)** takes out lateral and ventral corticospinal tracts (motors) and ventral spinothalamic tract (sensory – light touch), 20% chance of motor recovery – most likely to mimic complete cord – but **preserved dorsal columns so proprioception vibration and deep touch** is ok.
- **Posterior cord** (v rare, good prognosis) – tend to just lose proprioception,
- **Brown sequard** (best prognosis) – hemi section of the cord.

Q7. *What is the ASIA scale for describing cord injury?*

American Spinal Injury Association Scale According to impairment:
A 0:5 None complete   (0:5 = 0 out of 5 power)
B 0:5 None Incomplete (some sensation / spinal reflex preservation)
C 3:5 >½ of muscles less than grade-3
D >3:5 ½ of key muscles > grade-3 strength
E 5:5 Normal or **radicular loss (best prognosis)**

Q8. *What kind of fractures occur at the occiput?*

Occipitocervical dissociation *Harboview* **(ligaments injury) classification**:

- **Stage I**: MRI injury to ligamentous stabilisers, alignment within 2 mm
- **Stage II**: >2 mm alignment changes on traction radiograph
- **Stage III**: >2 mm on static radiographs (death)

Anderson and Montesano three occipital condyle fracture types - **treatment**
- I = stable, impaction against lateral mass; comminuted - **collar**
- II = stable linear fracture with basilar skull fracture - **collar**
- III = **Unstable** avulsion of attachment site for alar ligament - **halo/fusion**

Q9. What kind of C1 spine fractures have you heard of?

Levine and Edwards Atlas C1 fractures: hyperextension = ant or post arch fracture, axial load with lateral bend = lateral mass fracture – usually 2 or 3-part fractures or finally the **burst** = 4-part **Jefferson fracture** = axial load.

Management depends on **transverse ligament**. Its compromised if ADI >**3mm** or lateral mass separation >**7mm**. **Treatment**: halo then test for C1-2 instability with flex-extension radiograph at 3 months (>3.5mm difference = instability) or fusion if transverse lig gone.

Q10. How would you treat an odontoid peg fracture in a 50-year-old?

Anderson and De Alonzo classification:
- **Type 1** (tip #) is also instability of craniocervical junction injury **Harboview** –flexion extension films needed to rule out instability
- **Type 2** high non-union in halo 30% can also ORIF
- **Type 3** (into vertebral body). **Treatment**: collar/fixation/fusion (all are options).

*Q11. **What is a hangman's fracture?***

C2 fracture traumatic spondylolisthesis (hangman fracture) 'Levine and Edwards' classification. This is a hyperextension injury and pars fracture C2 (slip is C2 on C3).

Type 1	< 3mm sagittal plane displacement and disc intact = stable = **collar 6wk**
Type 2	>3mm displacement and or angulation C2-3 disc = **HALO or fuse C2-3**
Type 3	As for type 1 with bilateral facet dislocation = **HALO or fuse**

*Q12. **What is atlantoaxial instability?***

Instability at the atlantoaxial joint, types:
- **Degenerative** - downs, Rh, or os odontoideum
- **Traumatic** - odontoid fracture, atlas fracture, transverse ligament injury
- **Paediatric** - Grisel's (viral / inflammatory), Rh, trauma
- **Congenital** - Morquio syndrome, Larsen's, skeletal / chondro dysplasia

Peg view: Lateral mass opening **>7mm** suggests transverse ligament injury

Lateral view: ADI (atlantodens interval) 3-5mm children, 3-5mm in adults = normal, >5mm suggests **transverse** ligament and **alar** and **apical** and tectoral membrane injury

*Q13. **How can you classify this in traumatic injury?***

Fielding and Hawkins classification:

Type 1	Transverse ligament is ok, rotation, capsular injury odontoid pivot, soft tissue injury
Type 2	Transverse ligament rupture, facet joint pivot (ADI 5 mm MAX)

Type 3	As above + alar-apical ligament rupture both facets C1 sublux anterior ADI > 5mm
Type 4	Both C1 facets sublux posterior (odontoid peg fracture)
Type 5	Dislocation of facets

Treatment: requires HALO or fusion, **type 2 or higher is a relative indication for surgery**

Q14. What kinds of injury occur below C2 (sub axial c spine injuries)?

Allen Ferguson classification *mechanism of injury classification*

- **Vertical compression** → endplate injury progression to vertebral body burst
- **Flexion compression** → anterior column compression
- **Flexion distraction** → facet joint dislocation
- **Extension compression** → failure of posterior column
- **Extension distraction** → anterior soft tissues fail then posterior under tension
- **Lateral flexion** → compression fracture → contralateral soft tissues fail

Q15. When do these fractures require surgery?

White and Punjab general criteria – all relative indications for surgery:
- Flexion-type injuries tend to be more unstable than extension
- Neurology
- Facet dislocations
- Displacement >3.5cm or sagittal plane deformity 11 degrees

Q16. How do you decide when a thoracolumbar fracture might require surgery?

Vaccaro - TLIC score, 3 elements, score of 5 or more = relative indication for surgery:

Morphology of the fracture:
- Compression   = 1
- Burst   = 2
- Translation/rotational = 3
- Distraction injury   = 4

Neurology:
None   = 0
Root injury or complete cord = 2 (lower score as less to gain)
Incomplete/ corda equina   = 3 (incomplete injury has more to lose if deteriorates)

Posterior longitudinal ligament on MRI:
Normal   = 0
Suspected injury   = 2
Definite injury   = 3

Q17. Why must we take extra care when operating on Rheumatoid patients in relation to their C spine?

* **Atlantoaxial** subluxation (in up to 60% of patients)
* **Basilar** invagination – look for the dens migrating into the skull
* **Sub axial** subluxation / instability – look on the lateral c spine radiograph all due to inflammatory joint laxity / destruction (synovial)

Q18. What are the causes of lumbar spinal stenosis?

1) **Congenital/Developmental** Short pedicles, large medial facet joint = dwarfs
2) **Acquired** Degenerative changes with facet joint enlargement, thickening of the facet capsule, hypertrophy of the ligamentum flavum, herniated or bulging disk, loss of disk height, osteophyte formation (most common cause)

3) **Combined** Spondylotic changes with underlying congenital stenosis
4) **Postsurgical**
5) **Primary spondylolisthesis**
6) **Traumatic**

Q19. What types of spondylolisthesis do you know?

Spondylolysis is a defect in the pars interarticularis affects 5% of the population. 80% will be picked up on the lateral radiograph. **Meyerding Classification** is displacement relative to the S1 width in 25% increments from type 1-4. 100% spondylolisthesis is **spondyloptosis.**

Witse classification:

Type 1 (congenital)	- facets misaligned/ under developed
Type 2 (isthmic)	- defect in the pars
Type 3 (degenerative)	- loss of disc structure and facet joints
Type 4 (traumatic)	
Type 5 (pathological)	- destruction of facets / pars / pedicle
Type 6 (iatrogenic)	- surgically caused

Q20. What are the surgical indications?

Surgical Indications - pain after failure of conservative treatment and/or slip progression. For grade I or II slips, treatment is an in situ L5-S1 posterior fusion. With more severe slips, grade III or IV, surgery is typically a posterior fusion from L4 to S1. Slip reduction remains controversial and is associated with injury to the L5 nerve root (20% to 30%).

Q21. Spinal tumors, if it's a met or a primary is there any information in the literature to guide how you could manage these?

Tokuhashi score – greater the score more the indication for surgery, based on:

1) **General condition of the patient**
2) **Tissue type** – lungs, stomach, renal (poor), thyroid/breast/prostate (better)
3) **Neurology**
4) **Presence of metastasis elsewhere** (reduces score)

Printed in Poland
by Amazon Fulfillment
Poland Sp. z o.o., Wrocław